70 WAYS
TO BEAT 70

cx

70 WAYS
TO BEAT 70

Keys to a Longer, Healthier Life

David B. Biebel, DMin, James E. Dill, MD,
and Bobbie Dill, RN

a division of Baker Publishing Group
Grand Rapids, Michigan

Published by Revell
a division of Baker Publishing Group
P.O. Box 6287, Grand Rapids, MI 49516-6287
www.revellbooks.com

Printed in the United States of America

Library of Congress Cataloging-in-Publication Data
Biebel, David B.
   70 ways to beat 70 : keys to a longer, healthier life / David B. Biebel, James E. Dill, and Bobbie Dill.
      p. cm.
   Includes bibliographical references.
   ISBN 978-0-8007-3290-5 (pbk.)
   1. Longevity. I. Dill, James E. II. Dill, Bobbie. III. Title. IV. Title: Seventy ways to beat 70. V. Title: Seventy ways to beat seventy.
   RA776.75.B527 2008
   613.2—dc22   2008033113

Published in association with the literary agency of WordServe Literary Group, Ltd., 10152 S. Knoll Circle, Highlands Ranch, CO 80130.

To our mothers,
for trying to get us to eat our spinach.

Contents

Acknowledgments

We wish to thank Sue Foster for her research and written contributions to the manuscript.

We wish to thank Betsy Dill for her valuable involvement in this project.

We wish to thank Dr. Robert Martin III for contributing the original text for the chapter entitled "Save Your Skin."

The Voice of This Book

When we say "we" or "our," it means that we agree on the point in question. When we are describing our individual perspective or experience, we identify who is "speaking" in each case.

Disclaimer

Neither the authors nor publisher are engaged in rendering medical, health, or any other kind of personal professional services in this book. Readers should consult their health professional before adopting any of the suggestions in this book or drawing inferences from the text. The authors and publisher specifically disclaim all responsibility for any liability, loss, or risk, personal or otherwise, which is incurred as a consequence, directly or indirectly, of the use and/or application of any of the contents in this book.

Introduction

You want to live long; you want to age gracefully. And we want to help you do that.

But there's so much hype and hooey out there, it's hard to know who to trust or where to start if you want to "beat 70." Many people use supplements of one kind or another to try to slow the aging process, even though few products have any real science to offer in support of their longevity-related claims. It's not uncommon for baby boomers to show up in their doctor's office with a bag full of bottles and the question, "Doctor, which of these will do me the most good?"

In a broader sense, that is the question we tried to answer in this book. Of the thousands of products and programs promoted via the Internet, advertising on TV and radio, print ads in magazines and newspapers, and even whole books touting one thing or another, with ample "testimonies" offered as "proof," where does the health-conscious person start? This question is crucial, because with time rushing on and 50 *million* of your cells replacing themselves with each sentence you read on this page, you don't want to start down the wrong path if you can possibly avoid doing so.

Each chapter will show the health-enhancing, longevity-producing value of whatever that chapter's topic is. In creating the text, we reviewed hundreds of documents and visited thousands of websites, then summarized the best and most reliable information we could find, applying the "gold standard" of research as often as possible. The gold standard requires that a scientific claim should be based on independent, placebo-controlled, randomized, double-blind research. While anecdotes may be helpful in pointing researchers in one possible direction of inquiry or another, the testimony of one or even a dozen individuals regarding the health-enhancing effects of one thing or another does not prove that anyone else could or should expect similar results.

The challenge in selecting our topics was not, "How can we possibly come up with seventy chapters?" Instead, it was more like, "Which seventy of the hundreds of health- and longevity-related subjects will provide the average person with a reliable foundation for the pursuit of optimal health for themselves and those they love?"

We started with the conviction that health is far more than the absence of disease and that it involves far more than the biological components upon which many people focus. *Health* and *wholeness* come from the same root word, implying soundness in body, mind, and spirit. To these we added relational health, which has been shown to have an effect on longevity.

As one of our friends says, *health* is not really a noun but a verb, because it is dynamic, always changing as the sum of the relative healthiness of the factors just mentioned. So we tried to emphasize that the hope of improving our health is there for anyone willing to make the changes that will take him or her in that direction.

We focused on prevention as much as possible, since it should be obvious to anyone with an interest in health that the treatment of disease is *far* more expensive and distressful than preventing that disease from occurring in the first place. We hope that this conviction will continue to spread, not only among laypeople but also among professional health care providers. Fact 1: Most chronic diseases are preventable. Fact 2: Spare body parts are hard to come by. Those who are waiting for science to fix everything that they have broken or may break in the future are playing Russian roulette with their cardiovascular system with each new supersized meal they consume.

We also focused on simple alternatives, well within the reach of anyone who chooses to adopt them. After all, the basic principles of health really are uncomplicated. For example, Grandma said, "Eat your fruits and vegetables, and be sure to get enough roughage." Jesus said, "Don't worry." Mother Teresa said, "If we have no peace, it is because we have forgotten that we belong to each other." St. Augustine said, "Love God, and do as you please!"

The bottom line is that if you practice the principles in this book, you will be motivated and inspired and equipped to make changes that may be necessary. You will have a healthier living resource that you can trust and recommend. And you will have a scientific basis for practicing a faith-based healthier lifestyle.

In the process of creating this resource, we ourselves have been challenged and motivated to make changes in various health-related areas of our own lives. For we agree with Gandhi's exhortation, "Be the change you want to see in the world."

We are your fellow pilgrims on the way toward better health, affirming as we go that health and even longevity are not the true ends in themselves but a means to the end of fulfilling the purposes for which we remain here, with as much strength and vitality as we can manage, moment by moment, day by day.

Dave, Jim, and Bobbie

1

Accept Your Mortality

I don't want to achieve immortality through my work. I want to achieve it through not dying.

Woody Allen

Nobody wants to die, but by the time we're old enough to realize that "dead" means our pet cat won't be with us anymore, we begin to come to grips with the fact that everything and everyone will eventually die, including us. As much as anything else, how we adapt to that fact will affect how we choose to live.

Many people go to enormous lengths to ignore, deny, and battle against the reality of their mortality. The first gray hair they see, the laugh lines that were not there yesterday, the "crow's-feet," and the various aches and pains all announce that they are in fact aging even though they may still feel very young at heart. The cosmetic industry and anti-aging products, for example, offer a little false hope that the process can be stopped, or at least postponed a bit.

Some people, usually younger rather than older, seem to want to defy death through reckless or "daring" activities, perhaps to prove that this particular rule of life does not apply to them . . . at least until one of their friends or heroes ends up in a casket. Others are so fearful of death that they refuse to think about or talk about such mortality-related issues as making a will, purchasing a cemetery plot, or planning their own or anyone else's funeral—or even attending one. Some have faith that someday technology will be able to restore life or to clone someone who has passed away.

Others pretend that death can be overcome. As Dr. William Cheshire Jr. wrote:

> The quest for immortality has placed its faith in all manner of emerging technologies. So deeply human is the impulse to immortality that futurist Ray Kurzweil's hyperbolic prophecy of uploading the brain into a computer and living forever in cyberspace has attracted a curious popularity. According to Kurzweil, "At that point the longevity of one's mind file will not depend on the continued viability of any particular hardware medium (for example, the survival of a biological body and brain). Ultimately software-based humans will be vastly extended beyond the severe limitations of humans as we know them today."[1]

Ordinarily, as we age, we come to more realistic terms with our mortality. An Ontario, Canada, study found, "Attitudes toward death vary, but often older adults are less anxious and more matter-of-fact about death. As they see others close to them die, they begin to accept their own mortality, and tend to speak more freely about death and dying."[2]

In addition to the process of learning by observation over time, a University of Florida study found that faith can also make a difference in how people deal with death:

As they approach death, the churchgoing elderly are likely to find little solace in religion if they had little personal commitment to God during the rest of their lives. . . . The study of 103 relatively healthy older adults and 19 hospice patients in North Central Florida, all of whom were older than 60, found sharp differences between people who are "intrinsically" and "extrinsically" religious. Those with an "intrinsic religious" orientation dedicated their life to God or a higher power and reported they were less afraid of death and experienced greater feelings of well-being than people who fit into the "extrinsic religious" category of using religion for external ends, such as a way to make friends or increase community social standing.[3]

As we mature and internalize the reality of our own mortality, it will change us, hopefully for the better. There will be a new level of peace and we will do things differently. We will understand that nothing in our world is permanent! The beautiful sunset, the colors of the fall leaves, the garden after a rain, and even that perfect sweater or new car are only here for an "instant," so we better learn to enjoy that instant while it lasts. As the poet William Blake wrote, "He who kisses the joy as it flies, lives in Eternity's sunrise."

Years ago Jim and Bobbie were privileged to meet Robertson McQuilken, who was then president of Columbia Bible College. He has touched many lives as he shared his love for God and his own life journey in profound ways. That night he was speaking on accepting our mortality and shared a prayer he had written about the fears many naturally have as we age. It is called "Let Me Get Home Before Dark," excerpted here:

It's sundown, Lord. The shadows of my life stretch back into the dimness of the years long spent. I fear not death, for that grim foe betrays himself at last, thrusting me forever into life: Life with you, unsoiled and free. But I do fear. I fear the Dark Spectre may come too soon—or do I mean too late? That I should end

17

before I finish or finish, but not well. That I should stain your honor, shame your name, grieve your loving heart. Few, they tell me, finish well. Lord, let me get home before dark.[4]

One mark of maturity is to face the future hesitant of the dying process yet confident that the One who put us here will bring us home before dark.

.... 2 ....

Attend a Healthy Church

Don't let worry kill you off—let the church help.

Quote from a church bulletin

Over the past several decades, research has been showing that attending religious services increases longevity. Dr. Hummer and colleagues reported that attending religious services more than once a week was associated with an additional seven years of life.[1]

A long-term study involving more than five thousand California adults showed that those who attended religious services weekly or more had lower mortality rates than infrequent attendees.[2] In another study, researchers found that people who attended religious services once a week had significantly lower risks of death from all causes compared with those who attended less frequently or never, even after adjusting for age, health behavior, and other risk factors.

Why is this? Are churchgoing and longevity connected because gathering with friends is comforting? Is it because church attendees practice more health-enhancing behaviors? Or because there are many opportunities to volunteer within the local church and volunteering is healthy? Or could it be that church attendance strengthens your relationship with God and that makes you healthier? It may well be all the above and more.

However, before you rush out to the nearest church in hopes of living longer, be aware that not all church experiences are healthy. For example, one of our friends and his wife ran up more than $10,000 in medical expenses (thankfully they had health insurance) as a result of the stress of trying to deal with various issues in their church over several years' time. This involved hospitalizations for both husband and wife to deal with cardiac, blood pressure, and anxiety issues. In the end, the only way this couple could regain their health was to, in the words of the husband, "excommunicate" that church and leave to fellowship elsewhere.

We could cite many other similar stories, but the point we want to make is simple enough: Regular church attendance may be one key to longevity, as shown by various studies, but regularly attending a church that is damaging your health may lead to an early grave.

What are the characteristics of an unhealthy church? A few things come to mind immediately, based on our personal observation and professional experience (a total of over one hundred years, counting all three of us):

- a judgmental or self-righteous attitude toward those who do not think or act according to that church's (or denomination's) "dos and don'ts," including rejecting those who deviate from the norm

- a lack of tolerance for those of different ethnic or socio-economic status
- an undercurrent of conflict in which parishioners are expected to take sides
- periodic condemnatory messages aimed at various groups of "sinners," as if the members of that church are holier than others
- guilt-inducing pressure to serve, give, or support church programs
- an emphasis on perfectionism in any of its various forms
- a focus on control or power of a small number of people
- disdain for health-related considerations, as evidenced by the average girth of the leadership or the healthiness of potluck supper food

By contrast, a psychologically healthy church is one that practices genuine love, acceptance, and tolerance. Such a group can be any size or any denomination; it can be located in any state of the nation. But the common denominator is the ability of the church as a whole to embrace those who are hurting, in recovery, or lonely, and allow them to feel the love of God. These elements are crucial to one's health. We have been created to be in relationship with one another, collectively worshiping God and serving His people. Belonging to a healthy church enhances our relationships as well as our body, mind, and spirit, and all of these can affect our longevity.

In a healthy church you will sense genuine caring and acceptance. You will leave the service encouraged and challenged, sensing that you experienced and worshiped God, not weighed down with messages that make you feel guilty. You will feel a hunger to learn more of God and be drawn to a study group or fellowship group. There will be at least some attempt to draw you into the life of the church through personal relationships.

Feeling at home in a new church can take time. But be patient. The wait can be well worthwhile.

Overall, a healthy church will have some focus on the health of the whole person—body, mind, and spirit. It is encouraging to see certain denominations taking official steps toward education and other forms of prevention.[3] In addition, parish/congregational nurse programs focusing on prevention and screening are proliferating in some churches.

3

Avoid Fad Diets

We need to change how we look at obesity, stop obsessing on weight and BMI and . . . redefine the proper clinical use of weight loss drugs.

Dr. Jean-Pierre Després

When I (Dave) asked my mother to help me start to develop this book several years ago by giving me her own list of "70 Ways," the first thing on her list was "Avoid Fad Diets." She had me in mind, of course, because at that point I was in a high-protein motif. In a way, I'm glad she didn't focus on my BMI (body mass index), for example, because I would have had to don four-inch spike heels to get my BMI below 30!

A simple Internet search lists hundreds of "diets," many of them sponsored by someone looking to profit from your loss—weight loss, that is. Wikipedia.com lists more than eighty. The main dozen or so, A to Z are Atkins, Blood Type, Cabbage Soup, Fit for Life, Grapefruit, Mayo Clinic, Mediterranean, Okinawa, Ornish, Pritikin, Scarsdale, South Beach, Weight Watchers, The Zone.

The reason these are still around, while others come and go, is that they all work to some degree, if by "work" you mean that people who follow them lose weight. But the real question is whether losing weight should be the central issue of any "diet" you choose, since we all know someone who has lost a lot of weight only to pack it back on, bite by bite, until within a year or three they've become more substantial than they were before.

I (Dave) am a good example of that, since once upon a time I lost more than thirty pounds via starvation dieting (I chose to not list that one above). For some reason, perhaps because I was depressed or very unhappy or just needing to prove something, one day I decided to lose weight. The easiest way to lose weight, without changing the exercise quotient very much, is to severely restrict what you eat. It was hard for the first few days, but then it got easier. Over time it became an obsession. I wasn't obsessed with body image, like some, just with not eating and with the bathroom scale, which toward the end I would visit several times a day. Evidently I needed to prove something, so I did. I proved that I could will myself to weigh less, all the way down to less than I had weighed in high school. But of course, when I started to eat again, it all came back, plus some more, which is still tenaciously hanging on. In fact, the other day I asked my wife if my T-shirt made me look fat. She said, "No, you *are* fat." "How fat?" I asked. "About seven months or so," she said with a laugh. Fortunately, she loves every inch of me, even if she can't get her arms all the way around me anymore.

You could follow a high-protein/low-carbohydrate diet such as Atkins or South Beach. You can lose some weight while following the Atkins diet, but later you'll probably gain it back. If you like beef, bacon, pork, eggs, cheese, and so forth, a high-protein diet can be very tasty. Millions would agree. M-mm good.

M-mm bad. When you eliminate or severely restrict carbohydrates, you ultimately experience "ketosis" from excess acids called ketones in your blood. (Acetone is a ketone, and you surely wouldn't ingest that!) Ketosis occurs when the liver is forced to make sugar out of whatever protein is available, instead of making it from carbohydrates. This is not healthy in the long run, for anyone. It stresses your heart and kidneys. And your brain, which requires carbohydrates to some degree, may be forced into the situation of consuming its own cells in order to function properly. These diets are also high in artery-clogging saturated fat and low in essential B vitamins, vitamin C, calcium, and fiber, since many of the natural sources of these, including vegetables and fruits, are ignored.

The Blood Type diet has little or no science to back it up, though people do lose weight while on it, because they are restricting what they eat.[1]

Diets built around cabbage soup or grapefruit (or even peanut butter, popcorn, chocolate, or ice cream) can work when calories are restricted, because the bottom line of weight loss is that when you take in fewer calories than you expend, you will lose weight. But we suggest that any diet program that has at its core one prominent element at the expense of the balanced nutrition your body needs will ultimately do you more harm than good.

The Ornish diet is one of the best, because lowering your fat intake while greatly increasing your intake of vegetables and fruits is the only dietary program, which, when combined with exercise and stress reduction, has been shown to have potential to roll back plaque buildup in the arteries.[2] The Mediterranean and Okinawa diets are among the best and easiest to accommodate in the Western world, as their foundation is whole foods and healthy oils, while they still allow for adequate protein in the form of fish and a limited amount of red meat.

As far as The Zone is concerned, this "diet" seems to tap into the private fantasy of so many to somehow emulate professional athletes, who often speak of being in "the zone" when they accomplish spectacular achievements. In reality, The Zone diet is another reduced calorie diet.[3]

Tufts researchers found that there was no measurable difference between the results of adherence to Atkins, Ornish, Weight Watchers, or The Zone. To summarize, then, all of the A to Z diets have something to offer. Some offer online advice and support, perhaps for a fee. Others, such as Weight Watchers, highlight the need for social support when you're trying to make big changes in your life—and changing how you eat is one of the hardest things to change all by yourself.

4

Avoid Infections

The spread of disease and the emergence of new infectious organisms are the unintended consequences of human actions.

Neil Osterweil, writer for WebMD

Infections have plagued us since the beginning of time, when with little knowledge or defense we were helpless in the face of terrifying epidemics that claimed the lives of many or left loved ones maimed and weakened. Hope was always reignited with each new medical discovery, such as when smallpox and polio were wiped out. We dreamed of the day when most diseases could be controlled or eliminated. Unfortunately, we have only to listen to the nightly news to know that such dreams were ill founded.

We no longer live in the *Little House on the Prairie* where all food was grown or raised just beyond the doorstep. The whole world is quickly becoming our farmer's market. Dr. Robert W. Pinner, director of surveillance at the National Center for Infectious Diseases, says, "We can have cantaloupe from Chile for breakfast, tuna from Thailand for lunch, and Australian lamb with Mexican asparagus for dinner. A contaminated product in a locale which might, a hundred years ago, have affected a few people around the place where it grew now can be distributed nationally and internationally and cause outbreaks around the world."[1]

As a result, the concept of a superbug hiding on our person and around our home or community is something we must learn to live with in this new era. Currently, the most famous superbug is MRSA or methicillin-resistant staphylococcus aureus. MRSA is a type of "staph bacteria" that has learned how to dodge our antibiotics and prey on folks who have weak immune systems or are ill. These bacteria live normally in many common places, including our own noses, usually without causing problems. However, if they find a good host, they can wreak havoc because, due to our overuse of antibiotics, these bacteria have learned how to outsmart our common medicines. MRSA infections can occur in any open wound or puncture site as well as the eyes, bones, heart, and blood. The symptoms will depend on where the infection is: if on the skin, a red rash, boil, or blister will appear; if in the lungs, a person could develop a cough.[2] If you suspect MRSA, you need to see a doctor *immediately.*

A doctor (we will call him Ben) and his family had looked forward to a vacation for several years and they were enjoying every minute of each day, swimming, biking, and walking on the beach. The last evening they were there, Ben and his wife were walking barefoot along the shore watching a beautiful sunset when Ben stumbled over a rock formation. He thought nothing of it until several days later after returning home; while getting ready for work he bent to pull on his socks and saw a large red blister covering his instep. Then he remembered that his shoe had felt tight the day before, but in the midst of the busy day he had ignored it. Remembering the little cut he had incurred on the beach, he went to the hospital to be checked. Within an hour he found himself in a hospital bed hooked up to an IV, still finding it hard to believe he had in fact contracted MRSA.

While we do have some effective antibiotics for superbugs, those who study such things warn of the day when the current bugs will also learn how to resist! Meanwhile, it is up to us to take charge of our own environment and stringently follow basic rules of cleanliness. Our dogs and cats are often our best friends; research even tells us that to own a pet is life-prolonging—unless they are harboring disease. "Zoonnoses" is the name given for diseases that are passed to humans from animals; the number of cases is growing each year. "They come from giant Gambian rats and fuzzy bunnies. They come from puppies and pythons. Whether the animal is friend or foe, it can carry dangerous diseases."[3] One fellow we know nearly died from a bacterial infection transmitted to him by his parrot.

Keep wild animals wild—for example, squirrels or rodents can carry fleas harboring the bacteria that cause the plague. We know of a doctor who lost a young daughter who had evidently made friends with a squirrel that carried this disease.

If you do have a house pet, keep regular veterinary appointments and follow these basic rules:

1. Wash your hands well after handling your pet or the litter box.
2. Keep vaccinations up-to-date.

3. Avoid rough play with cats or puppies.
4. If your pet scratches or bites you, immediately wash the area well.
5. Don't let your pet drink from the toilet bowl.
6. People with weakened immune systems should take special care to not allow a pet to lick them on the face or near an open wound, and they should never handle animal waste.

Bird flu (H5N1) is a major threat even to those who live in the United States. In 1997, the lethal strain of bird flu appeared in the poultry markets of Hong Kong, transmitting its infection from infected birds to humans. The bird flu experts published a joint report in January 2008, warning that bird flu is now entrenched in the poultry of large parts of Asia, Africa, and the Middle East. The virus has not yet learned how to easily spread from human to human, a dire circumstance that scientists are hoping to avoid.[4]

Don't panic; pray! And remember that God is still God, and He is in control of all things. Do your part to avoid infections and you and yours should enjoy a long and healthy life.

5

Avoid the Debt Trap

Annual income twenty pounds, annual expenditure nineteen six, result happiness. Annual income twenty pounds, annual expenditure twenty pound ought and six, result misery.

Mr. Micawber (in *David Copperfield* by Charles Dickens)

If "the love of money is a root of all kinds of evil" (1 Tim. 6:10) and can lead one into many griefs, then the love of "plastic money" and other forms of consumer credit to buy whatever we want, now, can also lead many to grief. And that it has. The Federal Reserve report on 2007 consumer debt in America, released February 7, 2008, indicated that "revolving credit" totaled $943.5 *billion* at the end of December. This total has been increasing by an average of about 5 percent annually over the past five years. At this rate, by the end of 2008, revolving credit will top one trillion dollars for the first time. "Nonrevolving credit" (auto loans and so forth) passed that mark some time ago, and at the end of 2007 stood at about $1.57 trillion. Obviously, many Americans are spending more than they earn.

With debt comes misery, as Mr. Micawber said. With misery comes stress and ultimately ill health—psychologically and physically, and sometimes spiritually and relationally. Although there have been few scientific studies to date done on the direct effect of debt on physical health, an article published on WebMD in 2005 describes the chain of health-related consequences from having more debt than you can handle. "In an Associated Press/ IPSOS poll of 1,000 adults taken in early December, half of all Americans say they worry frequently about their debt, many of them saying they worry 'most of the time,'" the article said. "Stress increases levels of the hormone cortisol, which can lead to or worsen heart disease, high blood pressure, diabetes, and even some forms of cancer."[1] Other results can include gastrointestinal problems and loss of sleep, plus "comfort eating," which leads to obesity. Thus it's not only the interest that compounds; mental and physical disease follow hard in the wake of compounding debt.

The feeling that you are drowning in debt, if it continues long term, will be detrimental to your own health and the health of your relationships, due to the unresolved stress and conflict that can arise if one party is hiding the facts or one is blaming the other for the situation.

Al and Donna had been married over twenty-five years when Al made some risky investments without consulting his wife. To further complicate the situation, he used borrowed money to pay the bill because he was confident, based on the evidence he could obtain, that the company involved was going to pay a significant dividend very soon and that the profit would more than cover the expense accrued to that point. Unfortunately, those dividends never came, but the credit card bills never missed a beat. Ultimately, the only way out was bankruptcy. This did resolve most of their debt, but it also overstressed their relationship as they gradually drifted apart and ultimately divorced.

By contrast, when both spouses view their debt as a shared challenge to be overcome together, they are halfway to the solution, which involves (according to a number of financial advice websites) the following steps:

- Set financial goals—related to where you want to be, financially, three, five, or ten years from now.
- Determine where you are—because the only way to get from where you are to where you want to go is to compute your assets and subtract your debts. This is your "net worth."
- Create a spending plan—a budget is central to this process. The Federal Reserve has provided a free guide, "Budget to Save."[2]
- Reduce spending—buy what you need for less. Engage the whole family. This will expose the children to fundamental finances.
- Eliminate debt—starting with your high-interest debt. List them all, then pay them off, smallest to largest, over time.

- Create an emergency fund—since into every checkbook some rain will fall, the suggestion is to set aside three to six months' worth of living expenses. Start small and build.
- Carry adequate insurance—one uncovered medical emergency can bury us financially. Other insurances are important too, including life, disability, auto, and liability.
- Invest in stock—historically, the return is better than a savings account. No-load mutual funds are a good alternative.
- Make a will—significant savings can be achieved for one's family, and significant potential conflict avoided among them, by the creation of a written will.
- Give—charitable giving is a good reminder that even though we may feel "broke" most of the time, we are still rich by the standards of most of the rest of the world.[3]

6

Be Content

But godliness . . . is a means of great gain when accompanied by contentment.

1 Timothy 6:6 NASB

We yearn for the comfort and rest that comes with contentment. But we live in a society that constantly tries to make us believe that we actually need to buy that new car or new computer or wide-screen high-definition TV. Or maybe we need to update our wardrobe, because the media has convinced us that "clothes make the man," and wearing last year's styles is simply not acceptable. Salespeople try to convince us that an excursion to an exotic destination will fulfill our dreams and make us content. When we move into a new home we may be content for a while, but then we focus on the look of our old furniture and realize it does not fit in well, and our "contented feelings" begin to slip away.

Contentment and longevity are linked. In a study of 180 Catholic nuns, joy and contentment were strongly correlated with longevity. Contentment along with other positive emotions like gratitude, hope, and relief "may have the potential to reduce stress on the cardiovascular system even in the face of inevitable negative life events. Events arousing negative affect are approached with confidence that the future holds something positive and better."[1] On the other hand, if an individual's response pattern entails sustained negative emotions (or equally destructive suppression of emotion), the cardiovascular system can eventually be damaged. So, if your theme song is "I Can't Get No Satisfaction" by the Rolling Stones, you'll probably die younger than you might if you could learn the secret of contentment.

"I have learned to be content whatever the circumstances," the apostle Paul wrote from prison, with execution looming. "I know what it is to be in need, and I know what it is to have plenty. I have learned the secret of being content in any and every situation, whether well fed or hungry, whether living in plenty or in want. I can do everything through him who gives me strength" (Phil. 4:11–13).

Tim, a doctor, and his wife, Beth, were excitedly looking forward to getting into practice so they could finally have all the things they had waited so long to afford. The long years of scrimping and saving to get through medical school and residency were finally behind them. So they bought their dream house—a large five-bedroom home with a swimming pool in a beautiful area not far from the hospital. They envisioned a place where they would live happily ever after with their two daughters. However, Tim soon became enmeshed in the busy practice and Beth was swept up in the children's activities and community projects. By the end of the year their marriage was in trouble and their heaven on earth shattered. Then they both became followers of Christ and began to experience true joy and contentment that had nothing to do with their many possessions. They learned to base their expectations upon their needs, not their wants. Before long they had simplified their lifestyle and made a commitment to stay as free as possible from the debt trap and "conspicuous consumerism."

Contentment is more than satisfaction with something we've achieved, our relative fame or fortune, or the overall life situation we believe we have created for ourselves and those we care about. Contentment is a settled attitude of the heart—*an attitude that is possible no matter what our circumstances may be.*

Based on what the apostle Paul wrote about it, contentment may not be as much a miracle as it is a secret of faith that can be learned. Even Paul did not always know this secret. Earlier in his life, the apostle Paul was likely quite discontent. He was a member of a holier-than-thou group called the Pharisees, whose name came from the word *separated*; such groups often have a strong sense of competition regarding who is the holiest of the holiest. Paul's credentials were impeccable: "If anyone else has a mind to put confidence in the flesh, I far more: circumcised the eighth day, of the nation of Israel, of the tribe of Benjamin, a Hebrew of Hebrews; as to the Law, a Pharisee; as to zeal, a persecutor of the church; as to the righteousness which is in the Law, found blameless" (Phil. 3:4–6 NASB).

Even with such credentials, Paul had come to count all his human accomplishments as "rubbish" (the actual word used is far stronger, translated "dung" in the King James Version) compared to knowing the real secret of the ages—which is found not in quantum physics or any philosophy or idea, but in knowing and loving and serving a person named Jesus. From Jesus, Paul had learned that life was not about Paul but about loving God with his whole heart, soul, mind, and strength, and his neighbor as himself. As long as he was confident that he was seeking to fulfill that mission, he could be content, period. As Dante wrote, "In His will is our peace."

7

Be Kind to Your GI Tract

Never ignore a gut feeling, but never believe that it's enough.

Robert Heller

Few of us pay enough attention to our GI (gastrointestinal) tract, and even fewer treat it kindly enough. We take extraordinary efforts to cleanse and pamper our skin but treat our GI tract as if it were indestructible!

Your GI tract is made up of three major parts: upper GI tract, lower GI tract, and accessory organs. The upper and lower tracts are around thirty feet long and are like a railway system that runs through the center of your body, performing extraordinary tasks. The next time you go to the hardware store, check out the twenty-five-foot-long garden hoses if you want to get a visual of this system. The major functions of the GI tract are taking in food, digesting it, absorbing nutrients and energy, and then expelling the leftover waste. To accomplish these amazing feats takes a complex network of tubes, organs, enzymes, hormones, storage bins, and transit systems. Here's the incredible voyage of a Big Mac:

1. That bite of juicy burger is first attacked by a strong set of teeth breaking it down with the help of salivary glands and tongue.
2. Next it is thrust into the esophagus and, with the help of strong muscles (peristalsis), is sent to the next work area, the stomach.
3. The stomach churns the food into a liquid, adding various chemicals to break it down further, preparing it for the next part of the trip.
4. The small intestine is like an underground tunnel lined with an amazing array of small projections called villi that absorb nutrients and then pass what is left to the large intestine.
5. The large intestine removes additional water and stores the material until it is time to expel it.

With such a complicated process going on day by day, there is ample opportunity for GI tract malfunction. In fact, according to the medical diagnostic manual there are about fifty-five disorders[1] that can cause GI tract misery, including one of the most common, "irritable bowel syndrome" (IBS), which affects up to 20 percent of the U.S. population.[2]

Susan was thirty-five years old when she noticed during stressful times that she would have to rush to the restroom six or eight times a day. As if that weren't enough, she also had abdominal pain and bloating. Becoming more afraid to leave home and fearing she had cancer, she went to the doctor, who ordered a series of tests to determine the cause of her symptoms.

She was relieved when her colonoscopy showed no growths but concerned when she learned she had IBS. While there is no cure for IBS, much can be done to alleviate the bothersome symptoms. The disorder is complex and involves a disturbance in the interaction between the intestines, the brain, and the autonomic nervous system.[3]

If you keep your GI tract "happy," it will serve you well and for many years. Here are some tips for maintaining GI tract health:

- Don't put your GI system on overload with too much alcohol or additives—or even too much food!
- Visit your doctor if you have constipation or diarrhea.
- Feast on fiber (if you have IBS, follow your doctor's advice).
- Drink plenty of water.
- Manage your stress well—prolonged stress can injure your GI tract.
- Support your friendly gut bacteria with probiotics.[4]
- Wash your hands often to minimize ingestion of harmful bacteria.
- Eat fresh, clean, healthy foods to nourish your insides.
- Don't start a fire inside—avoid chili peppers and wasabi.
- Be aware that some medicines can cause irritation and GI bleeding, the most common symptom being black stools.
- Avoid "bad fats," which upset the delicate balance of your GI tract.

Please do not abuse your GI tract with unproven, dangerous myths designed to sell a product. Some well-meaning "experts" recommend archaic practices such as harsh irrigations and cleansing products borrowed from folklore. Others make untrue diagnoses of "parasites" and recommend products to "kill" them.

Most GI diseases can be easily spotted with the use of endoscopy, in which a small flexible tube is inserted into the upper or lower tract after sedation is given. A tiny video chip is attached to the tube, which allows your gastroenterologist to examine the walls of the GI tract for problems. This amazing technology is undergoing revision constantly, and new gadgets are being invented to make testing even more patient-friendly and less invasive. One of the newest stars in the field is the "smart pill," a diagnostic device about the size of a vitamin pill. Two types have recently been invented and should soon be more widely available. The first type houses a tiny camera and, when swallowed, takes thousands of pictures as it tumbles through the GI tract. The second contains sensors and a radio transponder and is able to transmit vital information about GI function, such as temperature, acidity, and pressure.

Your GI tract deserves a high place on your "care list." Treating it kindly will increase your chances of living out your later years without the burden of one of those fifty-five conditions.

8

Be Thankful

Gratitude . . . turns chaos to order, confusion to clarity. . . . It can turn a meal into a feast, a house into a home, a stranger into a friend.

Melody Beattie

Gratitude is a present-tense experience, a genuine, spontaneous feeling that arises from deep within and often occurs within the context of a relationship. We may feel thankful upon receipt of a longed-for gift, or when our doctor successfully treats a devastating injury. We may feel overwhelmed with thankfulness as we contemplate the gifts God has given us.

A gratitude study by Emmons and McCullough referred to thankfulness as the "forgotten factor" in happiness research. "Science is a latecomer to gratitude," they wrote, "whereas religions and philosophies have long embraced it as an indispensable manifestation of virtue, and an integral component of health, wholeness, and well-being." They found that:

- Listing life benefits instead of hassles every week resulted in a more positive view of life as well as more time spent exercising. Also fewer physical symptoms were noted.
- Subjects doing daily "gratitude exercises" were more positive and more likely to report having helped someone with a personal problem or providing emotional support to another.
- Those focusing on gratitude instead of hassles reported better quality of sleep as well as longer hours of sleep. Optimism and a sense of connectedness also resulted.
- Participants who kept gratitude lists were more likely to make progress toward important goals (academic, interpersonal, and health related) over a two-month period.[1]

True gratitude does not involve a sense of indebtedness—in other words, now that I've received something for which I'm grateful, I am indebted to the other to repay in some way. In fact, indebtedness erases gratitude, since one does not have to be thankful for something he or she intends to repay. Researcher R. A. Emmons reports that people with a sense of indebtedness have higher levels of anger and lower levels of appreciation, happiness, and love. Obviously, indebtedness is not health-enhancing.[2]

Bobbie and Jim learned a lot about thankfulness a number of years ago during a potential tragedy. Bobbie, then in her early thirties, discovered a breast lump and pushed through the fear to make a doctor's appointment. The doctor was equally concerned and scheduled a biopsy two days later. A new Christian at the time, Bobbie lay in the hospital bed the night before surgery contemplating all that cancer could mean to her young family and three children, ages two to eight. The fear was palpable and sleep impossible until she picked up the Bible and "just happened" to begin reading in 1 Peter, which brought an unexpected flood of peace. Meanwhile Jim, at home with the children, agonized about the outcome of the surgery. God met him also with a promise from Psalm 30:5 (NKJV): "Weeping may endure for a night, but joy comes in the morning." This enabled him to rest in God's care, regardless of the outcome. The next day they both experienced the epitome of thankfulness as the surgeon announced that the lump was benign! Yes, they were thankful to the surgeon. But they were even more thankful to God, who had taught them through this experience that He is the giver of peace.

One well-proven technique for developing a thankfulness level is to keep a gratitude journal. This helps people to focus on the positive and to think about life differently, especially events involving adversity of various kinds. A friend we will call Bill describes it this way:

> Simply jot down anything you can think of that felt like a blessing to you that day. Perhaps someone spoke encouraging words to you. Or a song lifted you up. Perhaps the sun shone and that energized you. Perhaps you saw a prayer answered, or felt the lifting of your spirits when you read the Bible.

Whatever blesses you, jot it down in just ten words so that you will remember it later. If you do this for one week straight it will change your perspective. Once you begin to look for God's tokens of generosity and love, you will begin to feel loved unconditionally.[3]

Adopting a thankful spirit is a significant step toward a healthier life. The Bible admonishes us to be thankful and gives us many examples of those who exhibited this quality. Depending on which translation you prefer, the word *thanksgiving* occurs about thirty times, and the phrases "give thanks" or "give you [God] thanks" occur more than forty times.[4] Clearly, God values our gratitude, but since it can't be because it fills up something that is lacking in Him, it must be that He wants us to be grateful because our gratitude is good for *us*. Quite possibly, it is good for us because it takes our eyes off what we think we lack and forces us to focus, instead, on what we've been given.

An attitude of gratitude is transforming and health-enhancing and worth making a place for in our busy lives. Some people think, *Why should I be thankful when I have what I have as a result of my own endeavors?* This view ignores the true Source of their aptitudes or intelligence, indeed, even their life itself. We have the opportunity to make every day another day to be thankful to the One who created and sustains us.

9

Be Who You Really Are

Live in such a way that you would not be ashamed to sell your parrot to the town gossip.

Mark Twain

Integrity is a health-enhancing, but somewhat uncommon, character quality. Its root meaning is from the Latin *entire*, implying completeness, incorruptibility, soundness, or an entity that is undivided. A person of integrity has what has been called "an undivided self."[1] Such a person is who he says he is, keeps his promises, tells the truth, lives his life openly and honestly, and is totally trustworthy, primarily because he has a core set of values and adheres to them consistently in all he says or does.

By contrast, there's the purveyor of "snake oil," smooth-talking salesmen, and many politicians—anyone who is willing to bend the truth in order to sell you something or to get your vote. With such people we just know that if their mouth is open, they're lying. However, lest we sound too judgmental, the reason we say that integrity is uncommon is that most of us have been guilty of stretching the truth in one way or another, even if it is not our habit to do so; for example, being less than honest on our taxes, cheating on a test, plagiarizing someone else's material, or intentionally deceiving someone for whatever reason. Mark Twain, who obviously knew a lot about this subject, said, "If you tell the truth, you don't have to remember anything." People who tell lies may not grow longer noses, but they do live in a state of anxiety, always trying to remember what they've told to whom.

This and the unresolved guilt that can go with it, is hazardous to their health, not to mention their reputation.

The psychological term for the inner tension that comes when our core values or beliefs are at odds with our actions is "cognitive dissonance." If your beliefs are in conflict with what is happening, you must either change reality or adjust your beliefs in order to resolve this tension.

Applying this to the question of personal integrity, let's assume that you are sixteen, and you've been taught (and you actually believe) that cheating is wrong, but you have a quiz tomorrow in Ancient History, and you simply can't remember whether Claudius came before or after Nero, though you do recall that Nero burned Rome, because you have a CD burning program called "Nero" on your computer. So you decide to write on the inside of your shirtsleeve a few important names and dates that will likely appear. During the quiz, you use that information to answer some of the questions, and you manage a B-minus instead of a D.

What happens next? If you wanted to regain some level of integrity, your sense of guilt would impel you to report yourself and take the consequences. Rationalization, however, is a less painful short-term solution, because it seems to adjust your beliefs to suit the situation a lot better. *I knew that stuff anyway. The shirt was just a reminder,* you tell yourself. *Besides, everybody else cheats once in a while. And, really, what does knowing anything about Roman emperors have to do with real life?* The net result is that you feel less guilty and you are more likely to cross this particular boundary again and again. If you take it a step further, you may feel obligated to cheat the next time due to the injustice of anyone expecting a sixteen-year-old to know anything at all about the Roman Empire. In terms of your biological, psychological, and spiritual health, the net result can be very detrimental over time.

Bill grew up in a home where very conservative morals were taught and practiced. Nobody lied, cheated, stole, or even thought of doing such things. He watched his grandparents on both sides celebrate their fiftieth wedding anniversaries. Faithfulness and integrity were deeply ingrained. In his early adult years, Bill was a model of integrity, being elected as a deacon in his church at a young age. So, when Bill had an affair that became public, the judgmental attitude and rejection of his church and family weren't enough; he internalized the guilt and developed symptoms of severe osteoarthritis, which continued until he was able to internalize something even stronger—a sense of God's forgiveness, love, and grace, which gave him back a sense of integrity.

By contrast, Gandhi was a person of integrity. A mother once brought her child to Gandhi, asking him to tell the young boy not to eat sugar because it was not good for his diet or his developing teeth. Gandhi replied, "I cannot tell him that. But you may bring him back in a month." The mother was angry as Gandhi moved on, brushing her aside. However, one month later she returned, not knowing what to expect. The great Gandhi took the small child's hands into his own, knelt before him, and tenderly communicated, "Do not eat sugar, my child. It is not good for you." Then he embraced him and returned the boy to his mother. The mother, grateful but perplexed, queried, "Why didn't you say that a month ago?" "Well," said Gandhi, "a month ago, I was still eating sugar."[2]

Living with integrity means being who you really are—without pretense or dishonesty—because you have a set of values that control and direct your actions, no matter what. When there is this level of congruence between your beliefs and your actions, you will be healthier and happier, and you'll have a lot more friends, for sure.

10

Break Bread Together

Kids who have family meals with their parents five or more times a week are much less likely to get involved with drugs or other risky behavior.[1]

Ann Tom

"Close your eyes and picture Family Dinner. June Cleaver is in an apron and pearls, Ward in a sweater and tie. The napkins are linen, the children are scrubbed, steam rises from the green-bean casserole and even the dog listens intently to what is being said. This is where the tribe comes to transmit wisdom, embed expectations, confess, conspire, forgive, repair. The idealized version is close to a regular worship service, with its litanies and lessons and blessings."[2]

In olden times (when we were kids) most homes had a dining room with a big table, where the family gathered for a home-cooked meal most evenings. Today, in homes that even have a "dining room," the table is more often than not littered with unopened mail, unfinished projects, to-do lists, school backpacks ready for tomorrow, or laundry that hasn't yet found its way to the closet.

Home design is adapting to our accelerated lifestyles, as one website explains: "A few decades back . . . traditional homes had a small kitchen, but a fairly large dining room. Families were bigger and they sat around a table and talked while they ate. . . . [Today] kitchens are larger because we are larger. Dining rooms are going away as more homeowners opt to put in bars and islands in the kitchen that takes the place of dining rooms. With all the different forms of entertainment, very few families sit down at a table to eat. The family room is taking the place of the dining room and many people are installing entertainment systems in the kitchen."[3]

Even when families do "sup" together these days, instead of that old-fashioned home-cooked meal with all its wholesome nutrition, the relatively small group of people is sharing an extra-large "everything on it" pizza. Or they're dividing a family-sized meal laced with additives, preservatives, sugar, salt, and fat—often hydrogenated oil—purchased at a fast eatery, dished out on paper plates, and eaten with plasticware to avoid the inconvenience of dishwashing.

Convenience is king in a world where everyone is on the run most of the time, so while it may be easy to blame the "fast-food" industry for all the ill health that has resulted since July 7, 1912, when the first "Automat" opened in New York City, this phenomenon could not have occurred without the hearty patronage of a time-starved public. White Castle introduced the five-cent fast-food burger in 1921. McDonald's, the world's largest fast-food chain (as of 2006, the chain had more than 30,000 restaurants serving 52 million people in more than 100 countries every *day*), had its inception in 1940. But it wasn't until Ray Kroc bought the company in 1961 that McDonald's as we know it was launched. So great has been the impact of McDonald's in the United States, that in 2005 the company agreed to pay $8.5 million to settle a lawsuit over its use of trans fat, with $7 million going to the American Heart Association and another $1.5 million to public education. Before you applaud too loudly, keep in mind that in 2006, the company spent almost $2.5 million *a day* on traditional advertising in the U.S. alone, about 40 percent of it aimed at children.[4]

Getting back to the family table for some good home cooking may sound like a novel idea in this day of drive-through everything and no parent left unemployed. But there is good evidence that the practice of this tradition enhances physical, psychological, sociological, and even spiritual health in homes where faith is a matter of conversation around the table.

In one study, reflecting nearly a decade's worth of data gathering, "the researchers found essentially that family dinner gets better with practice; the less often a family eats together, the worse the experience is likely to be, the less healthy the food and the more meager the talk. Among those who eat together three or fewer times a week, 45 percent say the TV is on during meals (as opposed to 37 percent of all households), and nearly one-third say there isn't much conversation. Such kids are also more than twice as likely as those who have frequent family meals to say there is a great deal of tension among family members, and they are much less likely to think their parents are proud of them."[5]

Tim and Judy are very careful about their heath. They exercise regularly and count not only calories but also fat grams. They avoid fast-food meals and choose their menu items with care when occasionally eating out. To help them stay on the straight and narrow they occasionally used to eat "burgers" in what they thought was a healthier form; specifically, turkey and buffalo burgers. Thinking they had struck nutritional gold, they splurged every couple of weeks on a "burger meal." They even told friends about it, and before long there was a gang going along with them. Then one day as Judy was checking out recipes on the Internet, she came upon some nutritional statistics on different restaurant foods. She was horrified to find that a buffalo burger has 892 calories and 57 grams of fat, without the cheese. Turkey was not much better at 812 calories and 45 grams of fat. Needless to say, they skip those "burgers" now.

Instead of staying in the "convenience food" motif, always having to check every menu at every fast-food chain to avoid killing yourself or your loved ones slowly, consider a return to the family table and home-cooked nutritious meals made from scratch. If this is very foreign to your family, start slowly and aim for several times a week. Turn off the TV and have a real conversation for a change. You'll be amazed at how much healthier you'll all be as a result.

11

Breathe Clean Air

You go into a community and they will vote 80% to 20% in favor of a tougher clean air act. But if you ask them to devote 20 minutes a year to having their car emissions inspected, they will vote 80 to 20 against it. We are a long way in this country from taking individual responsibility for the environmental problem.[1]

William D. Ruckelshaus, former EPA administrator

Longevity and clean air go hand in hand. While breathing clean air will not, in itself, give you longevity, it is absolutely clear that impure or unclean air can cut your life short. Numerous studies have concluded that humans can develop everything from cancer to heart disease or asthma just by breathing unhealthy air day in and day out. In fact, you may have noticed that your family doctor has added a caveat to his or her never-ending admonition to exercise, exercise, exercise. Physicians now caution patients to exercise *indoors* if the air quality in their area is compromised.

The issue of air quality is very complicated, but the atmospheric chemistry of pollution is becoming better understood. The best informed sources say that lurking in our own backyards is a whole array of chemical and biological pollutants. These include ozone, carbon monoxide, sulfur dioxide, nitrogen dioxide, fuel exhaust, air toxins (HAPS), and a host of dangerous particulates or aerosols.[2]

Most of us assume that government agencies like the Environmental Protection Agency (EPA) are actively protecting us or at least warning us of dangers in our community. But the reality is that "the EPA standards fall short and are only now being revised. A 2003 study of summertime hospital admissions of seniors at eleven Denver County Hospitals over four years revealed that ozone increased the risk of hospitalization *even at levels that meet the federal air quality standards.*"[3]

Airborne particles include a dizzying and ominous array of aerosols, including viruses and chemical emissions, many of which become lodged in our respiratory tract. The larger ones usually lodge in our upper tract and are easier for our body to clear, but the smaller ones (less than PM10)[4] become stuck in our lungs! A fourteen-year study of ninety-five U.S. cities found that even short-term higher ozone levels increased mortality from heart and lung diseases.[5] Our children, whose systems are more vulnerable to air toxins, are also at risk. Researchers monitored air at 147 California schools and found that 109,000 children were breathing unhealthy air.[6] In 1993–94 several important studies reported on the definite link between air pollution and lung cancer and other respiratory diseases.[7]

Other air pollutants have also been linked not only to respiratory problems but also to heart disease. An inflammatory reaction is set in motion and then proceeds on to arthrosclerosis, setting the individual up for a heart attack. Diabetics have been shown to have higher rates of hospitalization when air quality is poor. Reducing air pollution is important for all of us, but especially for the most vulnerable members of our population: children, senior citizens, and those with chronic diseases.

A striking study was conducted by researchers from the universities of London and Hong Kong. They found that cutting air pollution in Hong Kong increased longevity! Sulfur emissions alone from cars were reduced by new regulations and the results were noteworthy. "Annual deaths in Hong Kong from respiratory disease fell by five percent and heart disease fell by two percent. It is now estimated that Hong Kong residents will live on an average several months longer because they live in a less polluted city."[8]

We believe that in order to make it past age 70 we need to pay attention to the air quality wherever we live. It is obviously impractical for everyone concerned to build their retirement bungalow in the deepest forest or on the highest mountain in order to escape this dangerous health risk. It is likewise impractical to just decide to remain indoors for the rest of our years. (By the way, indoor air pollution can also be a major problem.) Fortunately, there are workable solutions, and they involve becoming well informed, taking preventive steps, and being wise about our chosen location and activities.

A physician we know moved his family to the Southwest to join a new medical practice. By his third day seeing office patients, he grew alarmed at the high number who suffered from respiratory disease. He had never seen so many patients with asthma in such a short span of time. He soon began to develop a cough and nasal congestion himself and decided to investigate. He was stunned to find that the city was burdened by a very high particulate count, which put its inhabitants at risk for a host of diseases, including asthma. As a result, he became a spokesman for cleaner air.

Fiction: The quality of the air you breathe does not affect your long-term health.

Fact: Many locales in the United States have dangerously high levels of particulate matter in their air, threatening the health of *everyone*, minute by minute, day by day.

Fiction: The government is going to protect you from this hazard.

Fact: Only concerned and well-informed citizens usually address this issue. *Will you become one of them?*

12

Build Strong Bones

You can extend the warranty on your frame—muscles, bones, and joints—and live longer and look better. It's tough to get spare parts.

Dr. Nick DiNubile

Our bodies without healthy bones or joints would be like a house without a trustworthy supporting frame or foundation. As we age, our bones can become weakened and our joints worn down. We are most likely to notice changes in our joints first. Our joints are like hinges where movement can occur between our bones. Actual contact between our bones does not usually occur due to the cushioning of cartilage, lubrication by fluid, and joint capsules made up of membranes surrounding the joints.

With long-term use, the cartilage in our joints that was once smooth can develop surface roughness, which in turn can lead to joint pain. As this process continues, areas of cartilage can become completely worn away, leading to actual bone-to-bone contact, further increase in pain, and the development of inflammation. The pain is usually at its worse in the morning and may improve with normal activity. But vigorous activity can increase the pain.

As of 2007, the Arthritis Foundation estimated the number of Americans with arthritis or chronic joint symptoms at 46 million, as compared with 35 million Americans in 1985. The foundation stated that:

- Arthritis is one of the most prevalent chronic health problems and the nation's leading cause of disability among Americans over 15.
- Arthritis is second to heart disease as a cause of work disability.
- Arthritis limits everyday activities such as walking, dressing, and bathing for more than 7 million Americans.
- Arthritis results in 39 million physician visits and more than a half million hospitalizations per year.
- Costs to the U.S. economy total $128 billion annually.
- Arthritis affects nearly 300,000 children.
- More than half those affected are under age 65.
- Half of those with arthritis don't think anything can help them.
- Arthritis refers to more than 100 different diseases that affect areas in or around joints.
- Arthritis strikes women more often than men.[1]

Osteoarthritis is degeneration of the cartilage and bone of your joints. It is more common in middle-aged and older people, but injuries can begin the process at younger ages. Obesity is also a risk factor for osteoarthritis, as is a family history of the condition. If you have osteoarthritis you may have more than joint pain. Your joints may appear swollen or "lumpy." Your joints themselves may lock if there are cartilage fragments floating around in your joint cavity. Your joints also may be literally "creaky" or they may make a snapping or grinding sound on motion. If you suspect you have osteoarthritis, see your doctor[2] because there are several ways to treat this condition.[3]

Weight loss may reduce joint pain, particularly in the large joints such as the hips and knees. Exercising can strengthen muscles around the joints and increase flexibility while decreasing pain. Medications such as aspirin and nonsteroidal anti-inflammatory drugs like ibuprofen can help the pain and inflammation but may have side effects such as peptic ulcers and gastrointestinal bleeding. They can also increase the risk of heart disease in certain individuals and harm the kidneys. Acetaminophen can also relieve arthritis pain, but excessive doses may cause liver damage. Even normal doses with excessive alcohol intake can do the same. Joint irrigations with steroids and synthetic joint fluids may be helpful. With severe cases of osteoarthritis, surgery may become necessary, either arthroscopy or the more involved techniques including total joint replacement.

Another important bone disorder associated with aging is osteoporosis, which causes bone weakening. After the age of 50, less bone is formed or replaced than is broken down. The honeycomb-like spaces in the bones become larger and the outer layer of the bones becomes thinner. These changes weaken the bones and make them more likely to break.

Kathy finally reached the age where she could retire from her busy and demanding job as an account executive. She had looked forward to an active retirement with travel, volunteer work, and more time with her extended family, especially her grandchildren. One day while working on her flower garden she slipped on a patch of muddy ground and put out her hands to break her fall. She immediately felt a sharp pain in one wrist. X-rays revealed that the wrist was broken.

While putting a cast on Kathy's wrist, the doctor said, "Kathy, the fracture of your wrist wasn't the only thing we saw. Your bones look thinned out." At the emergency room doctor's suggestion, Kathy went to an orthopedic doctor, who ordered a DEXA-Scan. He told Kathy, "Your bones have a low bone density consistent with osteoporosis." He said she should increase her intake of calcium and vitamin D and exercise more; he then placed her on one of the newer medications for osteoporosis. At age 71, Kathy is now able to enjoy her dream of active retirement.

Osteopenia is a milder condition in which a person's bone mass is lower than normal but full-blown osteoporosis has not developed. Osteopenia and osteoporosis can be diagnosed by a bone density test. A bone density test or DEXA-Scan measures how solid your bones are. It is important to have this test by age 65. The test should be done sooner if you have risk factors for osteoporosis, including a family history of the disease.

We are created with a wonderfully complex framework of bones. If we are good stewards of this important body resource we are likely to live a longer and happier life with more mobility and less pain and discomfort. If we take care of our bones we are less likely to suffer from the "groans."

13

Create Your Legacy

At 106, Jack Weil says he still goes to work at his western apparel company [Rockmount Ranch Wear, Denver] every day in order to spend time with his son and grandson, who have both played a role in running the business. What keeps him going, he says, is the chance to see them carry on a venture he built long before they were born. "I think I'm the happiest and luckiest guy in the world," Weil says.[1]

Our legacy is the gathering of the values, memories, experiences, perspectives, and accomplishments from those who walked the path before us. We then become the keepers of these gifts and the gift givers to the next generation. Our legacy includes our relationships, values, and accomplishments, all of which contribute to how we will be remembered.

One pastor's wife began the journey of creating her legacy after the death of her husband.

It came to me that I did not wish to be defined by material things or accomplishments . . . net worth, degrees, possessions. I wished to leave far more than that to my heirs. I wanted to leave a legacy in some form that defined to the best of my ability what I thought my life had meant, or at least some explanation of why I did what I did, how people and events have changed the course of my life, what things really mattered to me, and why, when I came to a fork in the road, I chose one over the other. I also wanted to pass on the wisdom I had gained through my life experiences. Most of all, I wanted to review my life for myself, so that when it came time to relinquish it I could do so with satisfaction and grace, resting in the peace that I had done the best I could under the circumstances, believing that life really is worthwhile and does make sense. I also saw this as an opportunity to continue to live life fully for however many days, weeks, months or years I had left; finish any unfinished business (forgiveness, reconciliation, put my affairs in order, things I still need to learn), embark on new adventures, and continue to grow in conscious awareness of all this. . . . I did not want to die with my music still in me.[2]

The awareness that we are standing in the space between the past and the future is a way of bringing purpose to each day. We are the keepers of precious memories that could encourage and direct the generation that follows.

When you reach age 50 or above you really become aware that you have already seen incredible changes—changes in your community, your church, your family, your way of life, the work you do, and perhaps in your values and beliefs. Part of your legacy will be in communicating what you've experienced and learned through personal stories that will be treasured by those you love.

Bobbie's grandmother, for instance, often told how God gave her an urgency to go to the bank and draw out their life savings the day before the stock market crash triggered the Great Depression in 1929. Those meager savings helped to provide for the family during the turbulent times that followed. Hearing such stories of faith helps to prepare the next generation for their own turbulent times.

We can create a spiritual legacy as we live our lives purposefully, praying for wisdom and keeping our eyes on the Giver of Life, while establishing traditions of prayer, Bible reading, and church attendance. God Himself is our partner in this endeavor.

Lee Wise says this: "Plan to leave an 'inheritance of great value' to those you love. All of us would love to leave a solid financial inheritance to those we love. But there's more: we can strive to leave them . . . the heritage of a good name; a strong spiritual heritage; a strong emotional heritage."[3]

Believe that with God's help you can "affect others profoundly, and leave a significant and important mark on the world while involved in what is meaningful and important to you. Each human being is endowed with talents and gifts that can make a difference and will connect meaningfully with someone along the way."[4]

It is helpful to actually write down the legacy you intend to leave. Listen to your inner desires, hopes, and dreams. Look at your life space and identify what you are drawn to. How do you spend your time? Be sure to include your thoughts and feelings. Some legacies will center on family. Others will impact a broader group like a community project, profession, or a church group. Some among us will want to start a scholarship program or involve the arts by painting or writing as part of our legacy. For some it will be building a trust fund for children or creating an heirloom quilt. The most important thing about your legacy is that it is uniquely your own—one of those few things in life that no one else can do for you.

A tremendous sense of peace can emerge from knowing you have created a legacy and left your own fingerprint upon the world. Remember that creating your legacy is a process, or perhaps a journey, the main requirement being that you begin before the destination is reached!

14

Cry More

"Big Girls Don't Cry"—Number 1 hit by The Four Seasons, 1962
"Big Girls Don't Cry"—Number 1 hit by Fergie, 2007

Crying has often been associated with immaturity or weakness, which is why some think that big girls shouldn't cry. Evidently "big boys" shouldn't cry either. In 1974, Edmund Muskie, former presidential candidate, seriously endangered his chances of winning when he choked up during one of his campaign speeches.

But sometimes tears are the only way to really capture the depth of one's emotions, and to stifle them at that point would definitely not be good for one's health. Dave recalls that, after losing one son to an undiagnosed illness, he was told that his second son's CAT scan showed brain damage. The pain burst from his soul, towered over him, then crushed him, and he broke down and sobbed uncontrollably for some time. Looking back, although one witness seemed to view this reaction as a weakness, he views those tears as therapeutic and cleansing, and his opinion is that had he suppressed them, he might have gone insane.[1]

The shortest verse in the Bible is "Jesus wept" (John 11:35). Surely the Lord is a better role model than "Rambo." In fact, the psalmist and king of Israel, David, wrote: "You have taken account of my wanderings; put my tears in Your bottle" (Ps. 56:8 NASB). Evidently our tears are not just wasted emotion but are meaningful to God, as expressed in the words of the popular 1971 song by Gordon Jenson, "Tears Are a Language God Understands."[2]

Crying was God's idea from the start, since tear ducts come as standard equipment for human beings, who cry most often when they are sad but sometimes when they are happy. Recently, scientists have been intrigued by the chemical and biological mechanisms at work in the act of crying, which turn out to be quite complex. Tears are not just drops of saltwater but are alive with hormones, enzymes, and toxins. "Biochemist William Frey has spent fifteen years as head of a research team studying tears. The team found that, although tear production organs were once thought to be . . . no longer necessary for survival, tears actually have numerous critical functions."[3] These include:

- Tears lubricate the eyeball and prevent "dry eye."
- "Tears bathe the eyes in Lysozyme, one of the most effective antibacterial and antiviral agents known."[4] "Without it, eye infections would soon cause most victims to go blind."[5]
- After crying, people actually do feel better, both physically and psychologically, while suppressing tears makes them feel worse.[6]
- Stress-induced tears remove toxic substances from the body.[7]
- "It is clear that crying is a primary way for the body to eliminate harmful stress hormones."[8] "During the last decade, stress hormones have been shown to cause serious damage to brain cells. . . . Unfortunately, stress hormones attack the very brain sites that are implicated in the perpetuation of mood disorders."[9]
- Tears enhance a sense of community by "deepening involvement in the welfare of others."[10]

Women cry differently and more often than men. Usually, men cry quietly but women cry with gusto, tears streaming down their faces. In *The Language of Tears*, Jeffrey Kottler, PhD, said that women may need to cry to get rid of excess lactation hormones. Women have been accused of using tears to manipulate, but in their defense we would suggest that crying can be a legitimate form of communication. The same is true for men.

Dr. Tom Lutz wrote that although tears were once seen as a sign of emotional instability in men, they are now considered to be proof that a particular man has feelings, and that he's strong enough to show deep emotion.[11] We saw this in future pro football hall-of-famer, Brett Favre, when he announced, through his tears, his retirement in early 2008.

An anonymous author wrote, in the magazine *Men's Health*,

I was worried about my inability to cry under any circumstances whatsoever. . . . So . . . I went into the kitchen, yanked out a bag of onions, and started peeling. . . . [B]efore I knew it, a veritable cataract of tears was cascading down my cheeks. . . . In my next life, I'm going to get myself reborn into an ethnic group that actually has emotions. . . . When I asked [Dr. Kottler] if perhaps I couldn't cry because I was getting older and my tear ducts were drying up, he said "no" without the slightest hesitation. "It's because you're a dour Irish-American." It was enough to make a grown man weep.[12]

Perhaps more often these days, men are weeping in private and in public. Former president Bill Clinton routinely sniffled openly. Former presidential candidate Bob Dole choked up while recalling how people from his home state helped him with his war injuries.[13]

Many public leaders, both male and female, allowed their tears to flow as a result of the events of September 11, 2001. This was progress, indeed. And by the 2008 presidential campaign, tears were no longer anathema. Mitt Romney teared up twice during his campaign in New Hampshire, and Hillary Clinton did so once. In Clinton's case, this seemed to help her win that state, despite criticism from rival John Edwards that the United States needed a commander in chief with more "strength and resolve." Edwards placed third in that state, then withdrew from the race a few weeks later.

15

Dance—Or Learn To

Dancing can be magical and transforming. It can breathe new life into a tired soul; make a spirit soar; unleash locked-away creativity; unite generations and cultures; inspire new romances or rekindle old ones; trigger long-forgotten memories; and turn sadness into joy, if only during the dance.

from AARP Health

Dancing has always been a part of American life. Our country's amazing melting pot has spawned dancers of every size, type, and color as they express their heritage. Some like square dancing, line dancing, ballroom, hula, ballet, tap, cha-cha, clogging, or—like Bobbie's grandmother—Scottish folk dancing. Bobbie has fond memories of Idie in her 70s and 80s playing the kazoo and dancing a little Scottish jig she learned as a child. "We could see the joy and exhilaration on her face as she relived the fun she had had dancing with her seven brothers and sisters," Bobbie recalls. "She loved to dance for the sheer fun of it, but the health benefits she gained helped her retain her strength and vigor well into her 90s. She embraced the old adage—die young as late as you can!"

The health benefits of dancing are numerous and can help

- strengthen bones and muscles and lubricate joints;
- tone your entire body;
- improve your posture and balance, which can prevent falls;
- increase your stamina and flexibility;
- reduce stress and tension;
- improve mental functioning;
- enhance psychological well-being;
- build confidence;
- provide opportunities to meet people; and
- ward off illnesses like diabetes, high blood pressure, heart disease, osteoporosis, and depression.[1]

Dancing, unlike some other exercise activities, can help the brain work faster and make new connections by combining music and movement. Researchers are studying the ways that dance is offering hope to those afflicted with Alzheimer's disease. Needing to memorize different dance steps and sequences helps keep our brains young. When patients hear popular old songs, they suddenly start to sing along or dance.

A dance usually lasts three to four minutes followed by a short rest; and if you dance for about forty-five minutes you are getting the optimum aerobic benefit recommended to strengthen your heart and lungs. Does dancing burn calories? Oh yes! Slow dancing burns about the same number of calories as slowly climbing the stairs, but fifteen minutes of fast dancing can burn as many calories as a runner burns in the same time.

Dancing enhances our social connections. Dance classes are great icebreakers, and many new friendships have been formed as newcomers laugh and learn together. Dancing fits the definition of the perfect exercise because "the best exercise program is one that is safe, balanced, promotes fitness and importantly, one people will do regularly because they enjoy it," says Polly de Mille, exercise physiologist at the Women's Sports Medicine Center. "It will result in the same health benefits associated with any form of activity that involves sustained effort in the target heart rate zone such as improved cardiovascular function, lipid metabolism, endurance and body composition."[2]

Those who have suffered heart attacks or have heart failure can benefit from slow dancing. It is one of the non-drug interventions offered to patients with good results.[3]

YMCAs and community centers as well as health clubs usually have dance classes, as do some churches. One church's aerobics class was recently highlighted on CNN—participants were exercising to Christian music, which uplifts them spiritually as well as physically and emotionally.

So choose a style of dancing that you think you would enjoy and join a class. Keep these general guidelines in mind:

1. See your doctor for a checkup before beginning.
2. Wear layers of clothing so you can stay comfortable as you warm up.
3. Begin with gentle stretches.
4. Drink plenty of water before, during, and after.
5. Be sure to rest between dance sessions.
6. Don't push too hard or too fast at first.
7. Check with your dance instructor to be sure of your form.
8. Sit and watch new dance moves first before you try them.
9. Perform regular leg-strengthening exercises.
10. Move as fluidly and gracefully as you can.

11. Cool down after your dance session, including stretching.[4]

Sometimes it is hard to believe that something fun can also be good for us. We are surprised to find that dancing can be just as health enhancing as sweating it out on the treadmill or exercise bike. Every hour we spend moving we can expect to add time to our life. Why not spend that time doing something we love. Dance!

· · · · · · · · 16 · · · · · · · ·

Develop Resilience

Character cannot be developed in ease and quiet. Only through experience of trial and suffering can the soul be strengthened, ambition inspired, and success achieved.

Helen Keller

As Henry Wadsworth Longfellow wrote, "Into every life a little rain must fall." Before our life journey is complete, each of us will face adversity in one form or another. Some people are broken by what happens, and they never recover. You might write their epitaph: "Died at 30; buried at 70"—that is, if they live to 70, which many of them may not. Why? Because when they were 30, something extraordinarily difficult happened—for example, a child or sibling or spouse died; they were sexually assaulted; they were falsely accused and imprisoned; or something similar—and in effect, they've been dying little by little, day by day, ever since.

Others bend and sway when the winds of trouble blow. Rather than break, they remain flexible and strong, and they bounce back. This is usually a process, rather than an immediate recovery, since most people need time to grieve their loss, learn and grow from it, and then accept and adapt to their new normal.

Those who seem to bounce back immediately may be saying the right things or doing the right things in order to gain approval from others, whether family or friends, or even from God. This is common in churches that teach their members that they should always be "up" and never "down," joyful in all circumstances, and even thankful for them too. False resilience of this type often results in some kind of emotional, spiritual, physical, or sociological disintegration later, possibly decades later.

Resilient people are not just strong, independent types. They are willing to express their emotions and to reach out to others, both in their period of adjustment, and later, in an effort to share what they've learned with others facing similar difficulties.

Resilient people tend to adapt more easily to change and to be more optimistic than pessimistic. They don't give up easily, and they maintain hope even when it's difficult. Despite their difficulties, they can see the humor in situations. They handle uncertainty better than others and they like challenges.[1]

The Resiliency Center reports, "Longevity research is showing that adults with psychological resilience age more slowly, live longer, and enjoy better health. A strong inner spirit can carry an aging body a long ways."[2]

Donna is a dynamic 85-year-old who has outlived three husbands, has lost two children to suicide, and has watched her surviving children struggle with depression and bipolar disorder. Even though she has faced devastating losses, she has bounced back from each of them and moved forward. She has more energy than many much younger women. What has kept her young has been her refusal to feel sorry for herself, her passion for helping others, her strong faith, and her zest for life. Always an optimist, she never loses hope, even when life gets her down.

The Mayo Clinic suggests the following as you seek to nurture resilience in yourself:

- Get connected. Build strong relationships with family and friends.
- Use humor and laughter. Remain positive and find humor in distressing or stressful situations.
- Learn from your experiences. Recall how you previously coped with hardship and draw on those experiences.
- Remain hopeful and optimistic. Look toward the future and expect good results.
- Take care of yourself. Tend to your own needs and feelings, both physically and emotionally.
- Accept and anticipate change. Be flexible. Expecting change makes it easier to adapt.
- Work toward goals. Do something every day that gives you a sense of accomplishment.
- Take action. Don't wish your problems away. Make a plan and take action.
- Learn new things about yourself. Find out what makes you tick.
- Think better of yourself. Trust yourself to solve problems and make sound decisions.
- Maintain perspective. Look at your situation in the larger context of your life. Know that your situation can improve if you actively work at it.[3]

Most healthy people learn to adapt to changes as an ebb and flow of life. They may feel sad over the loss of what was, but they eventually adapt and adjust to what is. Resilience involves changing actions and thinking to match the new situation. When people don't adapt or adjust, they tend to live in the past and miss out on the reality of today, day by day, month by month, year by year, until their sad journey is over.

17

Discover, Use, and Celebrate Your Talents

If you have a talent, use it. . . . Don't hoard it. Don't dole it out like a miser. Spend it lavishly, like a millionaire intent on going broke.

Brenda Francis

Got talent? Many people think not. But the great news is—we all have innate natural abilities. They are gifts from God, given to each of us to accomplish our purpose in life. The parable of the talents, told by Jesus (Matt. 25:14–30), teaches that the more we nurture and use what has been entrusted to us, the more the Lord entrusts to us. But if, out of fear or other reasons, we bury our talents, they never get used and we also displease the Master.

A talent is a natural or special gift, a special aptitude or ability. Just as a car has an engine, we all have something unique about us that drives us. One key to finding fulfillment and satisfaction in life is to stop focusing on our weaknesses and trying to improve them and to focus instead on discovering our abilities or talents, and then developing and using them.

Quite often that sense of fulfillment or satisfaction comes because "at the end of the day" we've used our talents to contribute to something larger than ourselves, to achieve some goal, or to help other people in some way. Satisfaction in life is one key to longevity, perhaps more significantly among men than among women, according to a Finnish study published in 2000. The researchers said:

> We investigated the role of self-reported life satisfaction in mortality including all-cause, disease, and injury mortality among healthy Finnish adults in a 20-year follow-up study that evaluated the possible mechanisms of actions using multivariate methods. . . . In summary, life satisfaction is not only a desired subjective feeling but also a health predictor. The relations of life dissatisfaction to increased mortality and to adverse health behavior support its use as a cumulative health risk indicator. Life satisfaction could prove useful as a research tool, in health promotion programs, and in clinical practice.[1]

It makes sense that when you are using your abilities constructively and helpfully, you have an overall sense of satisfaction and a forward-oriented perspective. There's always one more project to develop, or one more person to help—in other words, one more reason to keep on living and giving. By contrast, people who are convinced they have nothing special to offer humanity may labor at a dead-end job for twenty or thirty years, then retire—and expire—not much later. One study found that the earlier one retires, the younger one may die.[2] One antidote to this may be to discover and use your talents, especially in your later years, and that would include those who are able to retire younger and healthy enough to develop and use those talents to become a change agent in the world.

"For most of my life I told people that I was not a creative person," Maddie said. "Comparing myself to the great artists, writers, and musicians in the world, I felt like nothing and nobody. However, when I stopped comparing myself to others and started looking inside at what I really could do and what I was passionate about, I discovered a whole host of talents and abilities. This helped me to realize that God really did create a unique and gifted individual when He created me. This has been a huge boost to my confidence, my satisfaction in life, and my ability to make things happen."

If you think you might have some special talents but can't really verbalize what they are, ask yourself these questions: What am I already good at—keeping things organized, repairing broken things, woodworking, painting, home decorating, arts and crafts, writing, singing, playing an instrument, cooking, keeping the house clean? What activities do I enjoy the most at work, at home, or in any social situation? What do others see as my talents? What excites or challenges me or gives me an adrenaline rush? What am I most passionate about?

Using your talents can add to your vigor and enthusiasm for life, no matter what your age. Remember that "Grandma Moses," artist and painter, started painting in her 70s. Prior to that, she did embroidery but had to stop due to arthritis in her hands. She probably never imagined when she started painting that her work would be in such demand (one of her paintings hangs in the White House) and would actually be worth a lot of money—one painting was appraised in 2004 to be worth $60,000. When she died at age 101, she had created more than 1,600 works of art.

Dave, for whom this is the sixteenth book with which he's been involved, hopes that his own future will be like that of

"Grandma Moses," who never retired (and probably never even considered doing so). "Though I don't know that I'll live to be 101," he says, "I do know that I'll never retire. There will always be one more aspiring author to encourage, or one more person to help, or one more book to write, until 'The End' is written on the final page of my own story by Someone else."

18

Dodge Cancer

The most dangerous job for developing brain cancer? Plutonium hat model.

Jimmy Fallon

The American Cancer Society estimated that in 2008 alone over 1.4 million new cases of cancer would occur in the United States.[1] Over 178,000 women and 1,700 men would be newly diagnosed with breast cancer, even though many of these cases could have been prevented through lifestyle changes. Obesity is one of the culprits. We recently learned from the American Cancer Society that "being overweight or obese accounts for 20% of all cancer deaths among women and 14% among men."[2]

Physical activity is one way to dodge cancer. "There is convincing evidence that physical activity is associated with a reduced risk of cancers of the colon and breast. Several studies also have reported links between physical activity and a reduced risk of cancers of the prostate, lung, and lining of the uterus [endometrial cancer]. Despite these health benefits, recent studies have shown that more than 60 percent of Americans do not engage in enough regular physical activity."[3]

A healthier diet is also a good defense against the Big C. In 2007 we learned that avocados can help prevent oral cancer, probably because of the phytochemicals they contain, which have the ability to work against cancer cells.[4] Produce high in vitamin C may help you avoid stomach cancer.[5] Further, "Studies have shown that piles of broccoli help stave off ovarian, stomach, lung, bladder, and colorectal cancers. And steaming it for three to four minutes enhances the power of the cancer-fighting compound sulforaphane, which has been shown to halt the growth of breast cancer cells."[6] The same article stated that drinking two or more cups of decaf coffee a day may lower the incidence of rectal cancer by 52 percent.

"Prostate cancer is the most common male malignancy and the second or third leading cause of cancer death among men in the West. The descriptive epidemiology of prostate cancer suggests that it is a preventable disease. . . . Prevention strategies being reviewed include dietary fat reduction, supplements, dietary intake of soy, green tea, and tomato-rich products (lycopene)."[7]

To dodge cancer we also must guard against exposure to carcinogens, the most publicized of which is cigarette smoke. However, there are other carcinogens we need to be aware of, since unless we lock ourselves in a closet (without pollutants) we are going to be exposed to numerous carcinogens every day in our normal lives. There are eight pages of carcinogens listed on the website of the American Cancer Society (www.cancer .org), with suggestions about which ones should concern us.

Other important preventative measures include getting routine physicals and screening. The colon cancer death rate has declined at its fastest pace yet over the last several years as we have followed Katie Couric's lead and gotten colonoscopies. While it remains the nation's number two cancer killer, the death rate has dropped almost 5 percent a year for men and 4.5 percent for women.[8] More women are getting mammograms and Pap tests (and a human papilloma virus vaccine has been developed). More men are being tested for prostate cancer. These interventions can save lives—maybe yours.

Sometimes people who have watched loved ones succumb to cancer assume that they will follow. Yes, genetics has some bearing on our susceptibility to cancer. The recent genetic information on breast cancer, for instance, has proven that the existence of the BRCA gene can lead to cancer. This, however, is not a death sentence. It instead allows close family members of breast cancer patients to be tested and take preventative measures. Having the BRCA gene does not mean a woman has inherited the disease, but it does mean that she has a much higher risk of developing breast cancer. She can then determine she will eat healthily, avoid heavy alcohol use, maintain her ideal weight, and exercise regularly. There is a strong support network available for those who have faced and overcome these challenges.

A young patient of Jim's is one such overcomer. At the age of 23, she bolstered her courage and went for genetic testing for the dreaded BRCA gene after several in her family lost their battle with breast cancer. She and her husband were terrified when the results came back positive: a 50 percent greater risk of developing breast cancer throughout her lifetime. She is a strong Christian and through much prayer and support from her husband, church, and family she elected to have a double preventative mastectomy. She called the week after surgery telling us she had perfect peace and a thankful heart that God had given her the chance to look forward to starting her family without being plagued with fears about developing breast cancer.

Fatalism can be deadly in terms of cancer. Some people think that if God wants them to have cancer, trying to prevent it is irrelevant. Instead, they should be thankful that God has helped modern science develop a number of effective methods to diagnose and treat the Big C. However, it is best to remember that while early detection and treatment are important, in terms of cancer, an ounce of prevention really is worth a ton of cure.

19

Don't Give In to Chronic Disease

Not being able to do everything is no excuse for not doing everything you can.

Ashleigh Brilliant

Diagnosed with a chronic illness? You are far from alone. "Almost half of Americans of all ages have some chronic medical condition, and among seniors, the proportion is more than half. Arthritis affects 32 million. High blood pressure is a problem for 22.5 million. Allergies affect 20 million. Some 16 million have diabetes. Heart disease afflicts 14 million. More than 5 million have asthma. . . . You are a member of a very large club."[1]

The multiple negative emotions that initially accompany the diagnosis of a chronic condition are normal, but there is "a village" available to surround and help you. Chronic disease and longevity are not contradictory! In fact, many people with a chronic illness attest that after their diagnosis they became proactive about a healthy lifestyle for the first time in their life and actually improved their overall health while learning to manage their condition.

The U.S. Centers for Disease Control and Prevention defines chronic diseases as "illnesses that are prolonged, do not resolve spontaneously, and are rarely cured completely." The last phrase is sometimes the hardest. We need to accept (not like or give in to) the condition but realize that often there is no cure. Instead, we find hope in the fact that we can learn to manage our chronic disease and live full, happy, productive lives in spite of it.

James May was diagnosed with arthritis and struggled to come to terms with it. James relates:

> When most of you hear the word cope, it probably suggests "to be on top of it, to handle things with great success." Interestingly, that's what I thought, too. But when I looked it up in the dictionary I found the word was defined as "to struggle, to defend, to encounter," and "to have to do." I liked those definitions; successfully working with a chronic illness does mean struggle and "having to do," even when everything in us says we don't want to do it. . . . For years I taught high school students, and their description of coping was "getting your act together." My daughter calls it "getting a grip." They all seemed to imply that someday, sometime, everything would miraculously fall in place—and voila—life would be perfect. For a number of years I thought that would happen. What I have learned . . . at my ripe old age is that coping is really just doing the best with what is happening in my life at the present time. . . . Doing the best is accepting the reality that there are going to be good times and bad times, happy days and depressed days, fun times and sad times. It is a belief that through it all we can keep going.[2]

Important discoveries give us renewed hope in halting and even reversing some chronic illnesses. "Overwhelming evidence from a variety of sources . . . links most chronic diseases seen in the world today to inactivity and inappropriate diet consumption. . . . [T]his review is to . . . highlight the effects of lifestyle modification for both mitigating disease progression and reversing existing disease."[3] Many chronic illnesses that are not in any way caused by lack of exercise or poor diet can, however, also benefit from healthy lifestyle choices. Dave likes this phrase: "There is no condition that cannot benefit from better nutrition."[4]

Accepting the diagnosis and getting early access to proper medical care for your condition is very important, but it also can be frustrating. The medical scene has changed radically and now our trusted family physician must be aided by many specialists as the explosion of medical knowledge makes it necessary to divide up the care. Often it is the family physician who first diagnoses your condition or suspects a condition that requires referral to colleagues knowledgeable about your particular problem. This in itself can be frustrating, since with all the "doctoring" and testing comes uncertainty that all the doctors involved are communicating with each other! Even the experts agree that "usual medical care often fails to meet the needs of chronically ill patients, even in managed, integrated delivery systems."[5]

Most of us want to know all we can about our newly diagnosed condition, and that in itself will relieve some of our anxiety. Accurate information is a vital first step for designing a tailor-made plan to deal with your condition. You need to know about the resources available to you, the latest research findings, and support groups available locally or online. But insist on getting information from reputable sites, since there is much inaccurate information out there that can harm rather than help you.[6]

The question of "complementary" or "alternative" therapies will come up relatively early in your attempt to gain information. Our advice is to remember that while mainstream medicine has much to offer and should be your first line of defense, many complementary or alternative treatments can help with various conditions. For a comprehensive view of such treatments, see *Alternative Medicine: The Christian Handbook* by Donal O'Mathuna, PhD, and Walt Larimore, MD.

Make your doctor your ally and realize there are many good choices for coping with your chronic illness. Keep your doctor informed of all the options you are considering or have tried. Listen to your body as you try various regimens. Become an expert on your condition and invite your friends and family to come alongside you as you chart your course toward better health.

An MSNBC.com report in February 2008 entitled "Even with Chronic Illness, You Can Live to Be 100" said, "Surprising new research suggests that even people who develop heart disease or diabetes late in life have a decent shot at reaching the century mark."[7] So don't give up, and don't give in. Make any lifestyle changes necessary, and keep on trucking!

20

Don't Smoke or Hang Out with People Who Do

The tobacco industry reports that it provides jobs for 57,000 Americans. This does not include physicians, X-ray technicians, nurses, hospital employees, firefighters, dry-cleaners, respiratory specialists, pharmacists, morticians, and gravediggers.

Author unknown

Every day we hear or see dire warnings about the dangers of smoking. Yet every day smokers can be seen and smelled everywhere! Smoking is a powerfully addictive habit, simple to start and difficult to quit. These are the facts:

- "Each year, cigarette smoking in the U.S. causes approximately 438,000 deaths and results in an estimated $167 billion in health-care costs plus lost productivity attributed to premature deaths."[1]
- "Up to one-half of all smokers will experience death or disability related to smoking. Cigarette smoking has been clearly linked to the most common causes of death in the elderly and contributes to the morbidity and disability associated with many chronic illnesses common in this age group."[2]
- "Our study is evidence that smoking is, for all but some exceptional subjects, incompatible with successful aging and compromises life expectancy even in extreme longevity."[3]

Smoking is so highly addictive that most new smokers are hooked within two weeks.

When a person inhales cigarette smoke, the nicotine in the smoke is rapidly absorbed into the blood and starts affecting the brain within seven seconds. The result is the release of the hormone adrenaline, the "fight or flight" hormone, which increases a person's heart rate, blood pressure, and restricts flow to the heart muscle. The smoker will experience rapid, shallow breathing. Adrenaline also instructs the body to dump excess glucose into the bloodstream. Nicotine inhibits the release of the hormone insulin, which is responsible for removing excess sugar from a person's blood. The result can be that the smoker is slightly hyperglycemic, meaning they have more sugar in their blood than usual, which may be why smokers think their cigarettes reduce hunger. Nicotine activates the same reward system as do other drugs of abuse such as cocaine or amphetamines, although to a lesser degree. Research has shown that nicotine increases the level of the neurotransmitter dopamine, which is a chemical in the brain responsible for feelings of pleasure and well-being. The acute effects of nicotine wear off within minutes, so people continue to dose themselves frequently throughout the day to maintain the pleasurable effects and to prevent withdrawal symptoms.[4]

When research showed that secondhand smoke can hurt those we live with and love, more Americans were motivated to quit at all costs. We were sobered to learn that "the National Cancer Institute estimated that exposure to secondhand smoke resulted in more than 10,000 annual cases of low birth weight (babies), more than 2,000 cases of SIDS (Sudden Infant Death Syndrome), more than 8,000 new cases of asthma, and as many as 1 million cases of exacerbated asthma."[5] In addition, secondhand smoke is a known cause of lung cancer, heart disease, and chronic lung ailments such as bronchitis and asthma. In the United States 38,000 deaths annually are attributed to secondhand smoke, plus over one million illnesses in children.[6]

Smokeless tobacco is not the answer. Chewing tobacco and snuff were popular during the eighteenth and nineteenth centuries, and now the practice is reemerging, especially among young men, due in part to the number of professional baseball players who have been entrapped by this habit. "The studies show that snuff and chewing tobacco also may affect reproduction, longevity, the cardiovascular system, and oral health. One group estimated that the relative risk of oral cancer in longtime users of snuff varied from 1.8 to 48 times that of its occurrence in nonusers."[7]

Some people are motivated by fear to stop smoking, but others do better when motivated by love—love for your family, your friends, or even your own body. When you talk to someone you love about quitting smoking, be kind and compassionate. This is a very hard habit to break. Guilt trips rarely work. Let them know that you understand how difficult it is and you will be there to support them all the way through. Let them know you are concerned about their health and also your own and the health of others in your home, so if they must smoke, they should do so outside. Love motivates.

Encourage them with the immediate benefits of quitting:

1. Twenty minutes after quitting, your blood pressure drops to a level close to that before the last cigarette. The temperature of your hands and feet return to normal.
2. Eight hours after quitting, the carbon monoxide level in your blood drops to normal.
3. Within twenty-four hours of quitting, your chance of a heart attack decreases.
4. Two weeks to three months after quitting, your circulation improves and your lung function increases up to 30 percent.[8]

········ 21 ········

Don't Worry, Since It Doesn't Change Anything

Today is the tomorrow we worried about yesterday.

Author unknown

Once upon a time there was a carpenter, so wise for His age that large crowds came out to hear Him. He used simple examples to explain much deeper truths. One day, on a hillside overlooking a beautiful lake, He said something like this: "Just look around you. You see the birds of the air, and the grass, and the lilies of the field. They have enough to eat, and they're as beautifully adorned as any king who ever lived. They have everything they need, and so do you, and for the same reason—because God in heaven knows what you need too. So why worry about what you will eat, or drink, or how you will clothe yourselves—tomorrow? Each day has enough trouble of its own" (see Matt. 6:25–34).

Despite such assurance from that carpenter, Jesus of Nazareth, we do worry, don't we? In fact, some have called this the "age of anxiety." A report published in 2000 was based on two major analyses of 170 studies involving 40,192 college students in the United States and 99 samples of 12,056 U.S. children between 1952 and 1993 tracking "trait anxiety"—meaning that a person is generally anxious, rather than experiencing anxiety about a specific issue or event. The report's author, Dr. Jean Twenge, said, "The increase of social problems and isolation, coupled with media reports of breaking news events, can produce real or anticipated threats of physical and mental harm that contribute to this increase in anxiety." She predicted that this increase in anxiety would have long-term societal health implications, including depression and abuse of substances and alcohol. "Research has found that anxious people have a higher mortality rate, most likely because anxiety has been linked to higher occurrences of asthma, irritable bowel syndrome, ulcers, inflammatory bowel disease, and coronary heart disease," she added.[1]

Keep in mind that this report was published only nine months prior to the terrorist attacks of September 11, 2001, which only added to the U.S. population's generalized anxiety. A three-year national study of 2,729 adults was conducted by the Nursing Science Department of the College of Health Sciences at the University of California at Irvine following 9/11. The purpose of the study was to determine the effects of terrorism and acute stress on cardiovascular health. They found that

> acute stress responses to the 9/11 attacks were associated with a 53 percent increased incidence of cardiovascular ailments over the 3 subsequent years, even after adjusting for pre-9/11 cardiovascular and mental health status, degree of exposure to the attacks, and cardiovascular risk factors. Individuals reporting high levels of acute stress immediately following the attacks reported an increased incidence of physician-diagnosed hypertension and heart problems over two years. *Among individuals reporting ongoing worry about terrorism post 9/11, high 9/11 related acute stress symptoms predicted increased risk of physician-diagnosed heart problems two to three years following the attacks.*[2]

Worrying means to feel uneasy or concerned about something; to be troubled, to feel anxious or distressed. The word *worry* in ancient English means to choke or to strangle. In other words, when we're worried it can feel as if something has us by the throat and is choking the life out of us.

Almost everyone feels worried sometimes. This is especially true when we are facing situations that are new and frightening, such as making a move, starting a new job, going back to school. Feeling out of control, as with a job loss and mounting bills, can incapacitate anyone, even those with strong faith.

"I watched my father worry about everything, from money, to his job, his family, and the gophers that were digging holes to China in our yard," said Sarah. "My mother always told him to stop worrying and start trusting God to take care of us. Funny thing is that, after my father's death in 2004, my mother picked up all of his worries. She now worries constantly about her finances (even though my father left her well taken care of), the care of the house (again, it was always and still is, well taken care of), her very adult children, and those pesky gophers. Sometimes, I find myself worrying excessively about my income and mounting bills, even though I, too, am a believer. Although I have no trouble believing God can do miracles, I do sometimes wonder if He's paying enough attention to my current situation, or at least as much attention as I'm giving it."

Worry is a common response to life situations and life stresses. Excessive worry can lead to physical and emotional problems, even though most of the things we worry about never come to pass. As Mark Twain said, "I've seen many troubles in my time, only half of which came true."

On the other hand you might adopt the attitude of Scarlett O'Hara in *Gone with the Wind*: "I can't think about that today. I'll think about that tomorrow." In reality, worry is a waste of time and energy, and sitting there wringing our hands doesn't really solve anything. So Scarlett's approach may not be all that bad.

22

Drink Lots of Clean Water

Water is the only drink for a wise man.

Henry David Thoreau

Most Americans, perhaps as many as 75 percent, are chronically dehydrated, which affects just about every bodily process you can name. Without enough water, your body cannot detoxify itself or properly eliminate wastes. Dehydration can contribute to headaches, feeling tired and groggy, constipation, and dry skin—and even more seriously, to low blood pressure, circulation problems, kidney problems, immune system dysfunction, and various digestive disorders.

Adequate hydration, on the other hand, reduces joint pain, improves digestion, and may even reduce cancer risks. It is the cornerstone of weight-reduction programs. Your body is about 65 percent water; your brain, 85 percent. Your blood is 92 percent water; your muscles, 75 percent water; your bones, 22 percent. Water transports nutrients to tissues; lubricates; is the main component of tears, saliva, and mucus; and controls body temperature. You can live without food for several weeks, but you can live without water for only a few days.[1]

If you become dehydrated, a host of nasty symptoms will appear, including: mild to excessive thirst, fatigue, headache, dry mouth, little or no urination, muscle weakness, dizziness, lightheadedness.[2]

You've probably heard that you should be drinking eight to twelve glasses of water a day, but perhaps you don't really know how to quantify that. So here's a simpler approach: drink one-half ounce of clean, pure water daily for every pound you weigh, if you don't ordinarily engage in strenuous exercise (in which case you should increase your intake by about fifteen percent). Thus, if you weigh 150 pounds, you need about 75 ounces of water per normal day—about two quarts—and 86 ounces per strenuous day, about two and a half quarts. In warm, dry weather you may need more.

An April 2008 editorial in the *Journal of the American Society of Nephrology* calls some claims related to the need of increased hydration "urban legends." The article states: "There is no clear evidence of benefit from drinking increased amounts of water."[3] However, until further study of this matter is completed, we defer to the vast number of other recommendations related to healthy hydration, upon which our text is based, since dehydration could be deadly. Normal hydration is healthy, and overhydration is very rare.

One of our friends, a water scientist in a large eastern city, described the importance of water: "Water is important in chemistry, energy production, enzyme operations, nutrients, waste removal, and more. Water is the primary regulator of solutes (substances that are dissolved in other substances). It transports hormones, chemical messengers, nutrients, and salt. It lubricates the mouth and helps in the breakdown of food in the stomach. It is important in all the mucus needs of the body. It is important for lubrication of joints. It is important in the support of the spinal column. It is needed to quickly move energy and nutrients throughout the body when needed."

In America most of us take for granted that we have an adequate supply of safe drinking water. Recently, however, the Environmental Protection Agency (EPA) admitted that "all drinking water may reasonably be expected to contain at least small amounts of some contaminants." The statement adds that "the presence of contaminants does not necessarily indicate that water poses a health risk. EPA sets standards for approximately 90 contaminants in drinking water."[4] For the EPA's standard, along with each contaminant's likely source and health effects, see www.epa.gov/safewater/mcl.html. These contaminants include: microbes, radionuclides, inorganics, volatile organics, synthetic organics, disinfectants, disinfection by-products, and methyl-t-butyl ether (MTBE). Chronic consumptions of some of these contaminants above EPA safety standards can cause such things as cancer, liver or kidney problems, or reproductive difficulties.[5] In May 2008, a joint CBS/AP report revealed pharmaceutical contamination in nearly all U.S. city water supplies.[6]

The list of potential contaminants in our water, plus the assertion that *any* levels of these are harmless, has spawned a huge industry: bottled water. In 2006, the U.S. bottled water sales surpassed 8 billion gallons of water (31 billion liters), exceeding sales of all other beverages except carbonated soft drinks.[7] The total expenditure, in this country alone, was estimated at between $50 billion and $100 billion. We are drinking so much bottled water that the empty plastic bottles are causing a real problem in landfills across the country because "only about 13 percent of the bottles we use get recycled. In 2005, 2 million tons of plastic water bottles ended up clogging landfills instead of getting recycled."[8]

One solution to the quest for pure water is to install a filter on your faucet at home. Many Americans are taking that approach. Many companies sell filtration systems; the most popular brands being PUR and Brita. According to Brita, its high-end faucet filter system provides water for 18 cents a gallon, a considerable savings over bottled water.

You may find it interesting to know that water is used in the Bible to demonstrate many principles. Water is mentioned a total of 722 times from Genesis to Revelation. One of our favorite verses is John 4:14 where Jesus says, "Everyone who drinks this water will be thirsty again, but whoever drinks the water I give him will never thirst. Indeed, the water I give him will become in him a spring of water welling up to eternal life."

23

Eat Well, Be Well

I give you every seed-bearing plant on the face of the whole earth and every tree that has fruit with seed in it. They will be yours

for food. . . . Everything that lives and moves will be food for you.
Just as I gave you the green plants, I now give you everything.

Genesis 1:29; 9:3

In 2005, after many studies showed that the consumption of whole foods, including fruits and vegetables, is the true key to healthy eating, the government changed its RDA of servings of fruits and vegetables from five a day to between seven and thirteen servings a day, depending on gender, age, and level of daily activity.[1]

Healthier eating requires consumption of a wide variety of nutrient-dense, lower-calorie foods. The government's site explains:

> Nutrient dense foods . . . provide substantial amounts of vitamins and minerals (micronutrients) and relatively few calories. Foods that are low in nutrient density are foods that supply calories but relatively small amounts of micronutrients, sometimes none at all. The greater the consumption of foods or beverages that are low in nutrient density, the more difficult it is to consume enough nutrients without gaining weight, especially for sedentary individuals. The consumption of added sugars, saturated and trans fats, and alcohol provides calories while providing little, if any, of the essential nutrients.[2]

A nationwide survey done in 2005 indicated that even after years of pushing "five a day," only about 24 percent of Americans were actually consuming five or more servings of fruits and vegetables per day. About 36 percent were consuming three to four servings a day, and an even 40 percent were consuming two or less servings per day. This survey helped explain the rising tide of weight-related chronic illness and left no doubt that something had to change.

The Harvard School of Public Health reported, "The largest and longest study to date, done as part of the Harvard-based

Nurses' Health Study and Health Professionals Follow-up Study, included almost 110,000 men and women whose health and dietary habits were followed for 14 years. The higher the average daily intake of fruits and vegetables, the lower the chances of developing cardiovascular disease. . . . [F]or every extra serving of fruits and vegetables that participants added to their diets, their risk of heart disease dropped by 4 percent."[3]

Envision taking a stroll through the original Garden (of Eden), snacking as you go on a pear or a plum and some nice fresh veggies like sugar-snap peas and a spear of dew-covered asparagus that has just popped through the soil. Then you munch on some nuts or whole grains, with blueberries and raspberries for dessert. No "servings" to measure; no fats or carbs or calories to count; no additives or preservatives or trans fats; no herbicides or pesticides to worry about; no regimented meal times; no stuffing yourself until you're about to burst. Instead, you're just grazing along, with your hunger continually satisfied by the rainbow of delights the Creator has put there just for you.

In a broad sense, the simplest way to eat well is to make better choices, moment by moment, day by day, from the garden or supermarket to the table, both in terms of the foods you choose as well as how you prepare them. Keep the "garden grazing" image in your mind the next time you shop and expand your list of favorite veggies beyond what you usually buy. If the people for whom you prepare food are reluctant to expand their whole food horizons, try one new thing per week (or per month—whatever works). And if your loved ones' daily consumption of fruits and veggies is less than you know they need, you might consider whole food concentrates to fill in the gaps.[4]

We are what we eat. Our body can only build and repair itself and fight off disease using the nutrients we provide. And the real drama is played out moment by moment on a cellular level. If your cells could talk, here's what they might say: "Please feed us well so we can fulfill our part of your life dance as we were designed to do. We prefer slow food, no additives or preservatives, and as fresh as possible. And give us plenty of fruit and vegetable antioxidants to shield us from our constant free radical attack."

Your body has over 200 kinds of cells; between 40 and 100 trillion cells, total. While you were reading that sentence, roughly 50 million of them died and were replaced. Your skin cells will replace themselves about once a month, so an 80-year-old will have had 1,000 skins before he or she dies. Your blood cells replace themselves about every four months; your bones, every couple of years; your entire body, every five to seven years. So, if you feed your cells junk food for the next five to seven years, isn't it logical that your entire new body will be less healthy than it might otherwise be if you had eaten well during that time?

If your diet needs to change, purpose to change it—but take it little by little, step by step.

24

Enjoy a Hobby

Today is life—the only life you are sure of. Make the most of today. Get interested in something. Shake yourself awake. Develop a hobby. Let the winds of enthusiasm sweep through you. Live today with gusto.

Dale Carnegie

According to author Susan Sheehan, every hobby teaches you something. Her book describes how hobbyists and collectors all across the United States benefit from their pursuits. Often a hobby is what gives someone self-definition. Sheehan notes that people who are engrossed in such pursuits are often easy to talk to as well. "Their horizons have been broadened by their pastime and some have enjoyed extraordinary adventures."[1]

Dr. Walter Bortz, author of *Dare to Be 100* (Simon & Schuster, 1996), found that elderly patients who were active led more fulfilling, healthier lives than patients who weren't. "People who stay involved have a tendency to live longer, as they have more reasons to get out of bed in the morning," Bortz says. "Their interests stimulate their brains and this gets their bodies moving." He asserts that the brain, just like the muscles in our bodies, needs exercise—especially once aging begins and movement slows.[2]

Ted W. Mills grows roses as a hobby and is a rosarian and judge. In his article "A Rosarian Reflects on His Hobby," he writes, "Facing retirement, I longed for an activity that would provide both pleasure and a sense of accomplishment. In roses I found the satisfaction." He added, "Through all the trials and difficulties that I experienced at the outset, many blessings were wrought. Lasting friendships were made and I discovered that rose people were among the best of citizens. . . . All my industry became a labor of love as I shared God's creative beauty to the forlorn and ill among us."[3]

"Hobbies are great distractions from the worries and troubles that plague daily living," says Bill Malone. "Besides the reduction of stress and worry, hobbies can aid in the battle of depression. One of the simplest means to reduce the effects of depression is to do something fun and enjoyable. Think about it, have you ever seen anyone enjoying an activity that they have a passion for and be depressed while engaged in that activity? No, of course not. Individuals who are involved with their hobby are happier people."[4]

A study published in the *New England Journal of Medicine* showed that "mentally stimulating activities such as reading, playing cards, board games and doing crossword puzzles may prevent or minimize memory loss from the aging population." Malone writes, "The study compared exercise to mind building hobbies and found that mind building hobbies do more for preventing Alzheimer's or dementia than walking. If this is the case, let's play Monopoly, start the Chess or Euchre tournament before I lose my mind."[5]

We know the health benefits of an active lifestyle, so if your hobby is some form of physical exercise, such as swimming, walking, tennis, or skiing, you are improving the quality of your life in more than one way. An active lifestyle prolongs good health and contributes to an elevated sense of well-being. Recent studies have shown that staying mentally active may help to prevent Alzheimer's disease. So keep working on those challenging crossword puzzles, playing those board games, and reading, if this is what you enjoy. Those who challenge their minds at least four times a week are two-thirds less likely to develop dementia-related diseases than those who rarely challenge their brains.

Joining a stamp-collecting club, taking scrapbooking classes, or participating in an art class helps to fight loneliness and keep us connected and also helps to keep our minds alert. For those of retirement age, having a hobby can help smooth the transition from work to retirement. Scientists have long known that collecting things is a healthy endeavor, and collectors tend to be more social. Also, families that have an interest in collecting are healthier families. And collecting just about anything can be a lifelong endeavor, easily shared with family and friends.

Dave has had many hobbies through the years, but the one that has lasted about fifty years is archery. From bow-building to arrow-making to studying and using the technology that has so greatly advanced the sport over the past few decades, archery has been a great source of enjoyment and relaxation, and a wonderful stress reducer. "There is something magical, almost mystical, poetic, and even romantic about the flight of an arrow toward a target," Dave says. "For a moment, time is suspended as you wait to see the result. Perhaps this is one reason bows and arrows appear so often in films, and we never tire of seeing Robin Hood split that arrow in the bull's-eye. Thus far in perhaps fifty thousand shots fired, I've had four 'Robin Hoods.' Since the result is so rare, you just stand and look at it in wonder. And then you have to show others; as a result, the enjoyment of the experience is doubled."

25

Enjoy Your Work

If our work isn't mentally stimulating or emotionally fulfilling, it's virtually impossible to live a satisfying life. And a job that's overly stressful is just plain unhealthful.

Ben Kallen

Most people spend their early years preparing for the best job they can find, then spend one-third or more of their adult waking time working at that job, or commonly today, a series of jobs (some make as many as seven such transitions) until they retire. During much of that time, if you were to ask people who they are, they might respond by telling you what kind of work they do. Our work is important to us, not only because of the energy invested or the income provided but also because to some degree one's identity and self-worth are often linked to one's vocation. Thus, it should come as no surprise that satisfaction with one's job is a key contributor to good health and longevity. Conversely, dissatisfaction with one's job is stressful and unhealthy, even deadly.

Studies have linked job stress to back pain, heart disease, high blood pressure, and more recently, depression. "Researchers found that among more than 24,000 working Canadian adults, nearly 5 percent had suffered from major depression in the past year. Those under heavy stress at work appeared to be at particular risk, according to findings in the *American Journal of Public Health*."[1]

If you feel stuck in a work situation that leaves you dissatisfied most days, it may be helpful to know that about half your peers share your perspective.

> Americans are growing increasingly unhappy with their jobs. . . . The decline in job satisfaction is widespread among workers of all ages and across all income brackets. Half of all Americans today say they are satisfied with their jobs, down from nearly 60 percent in 1995. But among the 50 percent who say they are content, only 14 percent say they are "very satisfied." This information reveals that approximately one-quarter of the American workforce is simply "showing up to collect a paycheck."[2]

If you love your work, keep doing it. But in order to keep doing it beyond the age when many people only care to retire, you'll have to keep improving your skills and knowledge. A *Psychology Today* article, "A Day Without End," recommends:

- Broaden your career options. Pursue on-the-job training. Take work-related classes or training programs for different jobs.

- Maintain positive self-presentation. Be careful about personal appearance when at work. Develop a positive work reputation; maintain job competence.
- Reduce risk in health and job security. Minimize age-related risks to health and job security. Maintain a healthy diet. Avoid job-related health hazards.
- Continue professional/personal development. Develop work skills and outside interests. Read for new ideas. Pursue friendships outside work.
- Manage workload and resources. Reduce job stress by distributing your workload across time or to other people. Delegate work to others. Train others to help you.[3]

However, if you would rather "shove" your job than love it, take care to not "jump from the frying pan into the fire" by making a hasty decision to move from one employer to another, whose work environment may be less healthy for you than the one you're in now. Such rebound employments have about as much chance of success as rebound marriages. Here are some questions to ask yourself as you work through a job-change process:

1. If I had enough money to do anything I wanted for work, what would it be? Start with as long a list as you can create, then pare it down to three or less activities.
2. What additional skills or training would I need in order to successfully function in such a setting?
3. Where can I obtain the training I may need, or how can I hone my current skills?
4. Is there a way I can get some exposure to this arena of endeavor in my spare time?
5. Is it possible to make these advances within the context of my current employment?

The bottom line is that if your job is killing you slowly, maybe you should take the risk and try to find something that satisfies rather than drains you.

········ # 26 ········

Feast on Fiber

Ask not what your high fiber diet can do for you, but what you can do for your high fiber diet.[1]

Fiberlady

Grandma, the original fiber lady, said, "Get enough roughage." To her, that probably meant things like cabbage and broccoli and carrots and zucchini and cucumbers and potatoes, parsnips, turnips, and kohlrabi, and even celery fresh from the garden, various squashes and pumpkins, yams if you lived in the South, plus apples, pears, plums, and other fruits from the orchard, and home-baked breads made from whole grains. Sounds good, eh?

As early as 430 BC, Hippocrates applauded roughage for its laxative effects. The Bible lists the components of a high-fiber bread: "Take wheat and barley, beans and lentils, millet and spelt; put them in a storage jar and use them to make bread" (Ezek. 4:9).

It took until the 1960s for science to begin investigating the role of a fiber-rich diet in relation to health and longevity. As a result of forty-plus years of study, today we read, "Dietary fiber, found mainly in fruits, vegetables, whole grains and legumes, is probably best known for its ability to prevent or relieve constipation. But fiber can provide other health benefits as well such as lowering your risk of diabetes and heart disease."[2] Additional studies have shown that fiber helps conditions such as diverticulosis, irritable bowel syndrome, Crohn's disease, hemorrhoids, and even high cholesterol.[3]

A Harvard study of over 40,000 male health professionals found that a high total dietary fiber intake was linked to a 40 percent lower risk of coronary heart disease and a 40 percent lower risk of diverticular disease.

Joe had suffered from constipation for years. He suffered quietly, believing it had been passed on by his father, who also complained of bowel problems, especially as he aged. Finally, at the insistence of his wife, Joe agreed to see a doctor. He was astounded when he learned that help was available and that untreated constipation could lead to a horde of health problems. At the doctor's bidding he began slowly adding fiber-rich foods to his meals. Two months later he was elated to report that his constipation had greatly improved and that the extra fiber eliminated his between-meal hunger. In addition, he discovered that his cholesterol and weight were back in a healthy range. Joe's father soon followed suit, and as a result both men greatly increased their chances for a long, healthy life.

Dietary fiber is basically carbohydrates that cannot be digested or absorbed. Fiber, sometimes called roughage or bulk, is present in all plants that can be eaten for food. The list of sources of fiber mentioned in this chapter is by no means comprehensive. Fiber is categorized into two types:

Insoluble fiber—increases the movement of waste material through the colon. This is important because it will aid in exerting less pressure on the colon walls and keeps waste from reabsorbing. Insoluble fiber includes: whole grains (whole wheat bread, barley, couscous, brown rice, bulgur, whole grain cereal), wheat bran, seeds, carrots, cucumbers, zucchini, celery.

Soluble fiber—dissolves in water and forms a gel-like material that aids the body in a number of ways, one of which is to block the absorption of cholesterol. Soluble fiber is found in: oatmeal, brans—oat, barley, rice—nuts and seeds, legumes (dried peas, beans, lentils), apples, pears, strawberries, blueberries.[4] One site that lists the fiber in many vegetables and fruits lists black beans as #1.[5]

Most studies recommend that we get at least 21 to 38 grams of dietary fiber a day depending on gender and age. If you are consuming less now, upgrade slowly in order to give your body a chance to adjust. The following tips are based on a Mayo Clinic list:

- Start your day with a high-fiber breakfast cereal—5 or more grams of fiber per serving.
- Add crushed bran cereal or unprocessed wheat bran to baked products—meat loaf, breads, muffins, casseroles, cakes, and cookies.
- Eat whole-grain breads with at least 2 grams of fiber per serving.
- Substitute whole-grain flour for half or all of the white flour when baking bread. Adjust yeast or baking powder accordingly.
- Try brown rice, barley, whole-wheat pasta, and bulgur.
- Eat more beans, peas, and lentils. Add kidney beans to canned soup or a green salad.
- Eat fruit at every meal. Apples, bananas, oranges, pears, and berries are good sources of fiber.

- Make snacks count. Fresh and dried fruit, raw vegetables, low-fat popcorn, and whole-grain crackers are all good choices.[6]

27

Forgive Others

Forgiveness [is] the tofu of the soul, a healthful alternative to the red meat of anger and vengeance. In a way, the most selfish thing you can do for yourself is to forgive other people.[1]

Dr. Dean Ornish

Research suggests that forgiveness improves health because it "reduces the stress that comes from a state of unforgiveness: a potent mix of bitterness, anger, hostility, hatred, resentment, and fear. These have physiologic consequences including high blood pressure, hormone changes linked to heart disease, suppression of immune system, and possibly even impaired brain function and memory. [Forgiveness] allows those who are able to forgive to have better interpersonal functioning and therefore social support. . . . A large body of research shows that social support reduces cardiovascular risks, decreases recovery time and increases survival from several types of cancer."[2]

The spiritual consequences of forgiveness are equally crucial. Dr. Christina Puchalski, assistant professor of medicine at George Washington University Medical School, has explored the link between inner peace and health. "The act of forgiveness can result in less anxiety and depression, better health outcomes, increased coping with stress, and increased closeness to God and others."[3] Inability to forgive blocks hope—without hope there is no future. Dr. Puchalski cautions that unless we forgive we cannot feel God's presence.[4] Persistent unforgiveness is a trap of human nature from which we need God's help to break free.

Dr. Everett Worthington defines forgiveness as "an emotional replacement of unforgiving feelings with positive emotions, such as love, empathy, or compassion."[5] Lewis Smedes describes forgiveness in this way: "When we forgive, we transcend the pain we feel by surrendering the right to get even with the person who hurt us."[6]

Jim's mom, Louise, was working in her garden, enjoying a beautiful spring day when the phone rang. It was her sister-in-law, Hart, asking if Louise would ride along with her to the mall. One to never turn down an outing, Louise put her gardening aside and happily accepted the offer. On the way to the mall, while rounding a corner, Hart suddenly swerved off the road, running head-on into a telephone pole. Hart was unhurt, but Louise was pinned in the twisted front seat, her body encased in a metal vice. It took the jaws of life to free her, and as she was rushed toward the hospital with her blood pressure dropping dangerously low, she knew her life was going to be changed forever. Weeks and months of painful treatment and rehab followed as doctors fought to save her leg.

Louise underwent many surgeries and skin grafts. When she finally emerged from the hospital, she was weak and in pain and realized she would need a walker to get around for the rest of her life. But everyone who knew her was amazed by her consistent positive attitude and her total lack of negativity toward Hart. In fact, she was often more concerned for Hart's recovery from depression and self-blame than for her own healing journey. When asked how she could be so forgiving of Hart when her life had been so altered by the accident, she always answered that she had been in prayer and the Lord was taking care of it all. Louise, who died in 2007, spent the rest of her life often in pain and limited in mobility but full of peace and joy. She was an unforgettable example to her friends and family. Hart, now a widow and in a nursing home, received a phone call faithfully every evening from Louise until she passed away.

By contrast, some people seem unable to forgive; this is surely toxic to their body, mind, soul, and relationships and shortens their lives. Everett Worthington, director of A Campaign for Forgiveness, says, "It happens down the line but every time you feel unforgiveness, you are more likely to develop a health problem."[7] No wonder forgiveness research has become, in the past few years, one of the hottest topics in clinical psychology, tallying more than 1,200 studies thus far.

Forgiveness does not necessarily mean forgetting (as if we could), condoning wrong or hurtful behavior, or excusing the offender; nor does it mean we can never experience justifiable anger or wish for justice.

Forgiveness does mean deciding to let go of our own hurt, our own suffering, our own ruminating over grievances, our own plotting for revenge. For most of us, this is a process, not a solitary act. In other words, we may need to learn to forgive again and again.

In 2006, the world was stunned as a gunman entered an Amish school in Pennsylvania and methodically shot ten girls, killing five and wounding the others. We watched in horror as the events unfolded and then sat transfixed a few hours later as a number of the Amish community went to the killer's home to express their heartfelt forgiveness to his family. They did this because they believed that their faith hero, Jesus, would have acted similarly. Without doubt, it was a good lesson for all of us.

28

Forgive Yourself

To forgive is to set a prisoner free and discover that the prisoner was you.

Lewis B. Smedes

There is a great line from the movie *Toy Story* when Rex the Dinosaur discovers that Woody and Buzz Lightyear have been telling the truth, when Rex and the other characters thought Woody and Buzz had been stretching the truth just a bit. At that moment the big green dinosaur, an emotional character prone to panic attacks, states, "Great, now I have guilt."

Like Rex, most of us feel a sense of failure, resulting in guilt, when we have done or said something wrong, hurt another person thoughtlessly, thought ill of someone when it was unfounded, lied about something, taken something that was not ours, or worse. But is guilt all bad? Not necessarily, says psychology professor June Tangney: "People generally feel guilt when they've done something that violates their own moral standards. Guilt motivates people to make things right when they do something wrong. It's a helpful, adaptive way to feel bad."[1]

Guilt is a feeling of responsibility for having done something wrong. Feelings associated with guilt include regret, remorse, or feeling obligated to make things right. A healthy sense of guilt is what we should feel when we have done something wrong. An unhealthy sense of guilt occurs when we have done nothing wrong but feel guilty anyway.

A British study found that "people who feel guilty about life's pleasures may be damaging their health. . . . A group of volunteers were asked to list their most pleasurable activities, which included sex, eating chocolate, drinking, and smoking. They were asked to rate them according to how much pleasure and guilt they caused. They were also asked to provide samples of saliva, which were measured for levels of immunoglobulin A. High levels of this antibody are associated with a strong immune system and the ability to fight off illness. The researchers found that immunoglobulin A levels were lower in those people whose pleasures were accompanied by more feelings of guilt."[2]

Exaggerated feelings of guilt can negatively affect self-esteem and self-worth and lead to self-destructive behavior such as self-mutilation, drug abuse and alcoholism, depression, relationship issues, or even suicide.

Unresolved guilt can result in a variety of physical symptoms. Dr. Jim says that when you cannot forgive yourself and you don't feel forgiven, your body acts "guilty." Your autonomic nervous system is out of balance, alternating between symptoms stimulated by the vagus nerve and those stimulated by adrenalin. Over a prolonged period, some of these processes can damage parts of your body, producing such symptoms as insomnia, heart palpitations, heartburn (reflux), high blood pressure, abdominal pain, change in bowel habits, and headaches (including migraines). Because your autonomic nervous system responds more to your emotions than to your thinking, the symptoms usually do not go away until you actually *feel* forgiven.

Some people seem to feel guilty most of the time about most everything. They insist on apologizing for every little thing. They may struggle with low self-esteem, perfectionist tendencies, resentment, and an inability to forgive others and themselves. Such people tend to be laden with anxiety; they need to be in control. They sometimes exhibit symptoms of obsessive-compulsive disorder, or "panic disorder."[3] Quite often they have never recovered from a significant traumatic event, and many of their symptoms can be an expression of post-traumatic stress disorder.

"When my daughter died by suicide in 1991," said Sue, "the guilt I felt was debilitating. In my mind, I became the worst mother in the world, otherwise why would she have done what she did? A counselor told me that my daughter had forgiven me for any wrongs done to her, and I would be wise to forgive myself. It took me a long time to realize that he was right. When I came to accept that I had done the best job I could as a parent even though there were things I would do differently if I could do it all over, and that I was not the reason for her choice, I could forgive myself and then deal with the guilt in healthy ways."

The psalmist and king of Israel, David, described the effects of unresolved guilt, and the cure, as well:

> When I kept silent about my sin, my body wasted away
> Through my groaning all day long.
> For day and night Your hand was heavy upon me;
> My vitality was drained away as with the fever heat of
> summer.

Remember that David had committed adultery with Bathsheba, gotten her pregnant, then had her soldier-husband put in harm's way so he would be killed in battle. Even so, when David confessed his sin, he was forgiven and his spiritual, physical, and emotional health was restored:

> I acknowledged my sin to You,
> And my iniquity I did not hide;
> I said, "I will confess my transgressions to the LORD";
> And You forgave the guilt of my sin.
>
> Psalm 32:3–5 NASB

100

Since it is unlikely that what you've done (or left undone) is worse than David's crimes, doesn't it seem like a health-enhancing choice to confess your sins to the Lord, accept forgiveness, and then get on with living?

29

Fulfill Your Purpose

Living a life of purpose reflects who you are deep inside, your beliefs, values and passion for living. It is about following your heart and doing what you love to do with passion and purpose.

Tressa Ryan

Every new electronic gadget or appliance arrives with a set of complete instructions describing how to assemble it, use it, clean it, and get the best service from it. However, with the greatest "delivery" of all, our new baby, we may get a few clues about care and feeding but no operating instructions or even a limited description of intended purpose!

That is, of course, because our purpose is unique to each of us, and discovering and fulfilling it is one of life's most exciting, frustrating, or even challenging adventures. Yet knowing and fulfilling our purpose will determine the sense of meaning, satisfaction, and fulfillment we'll experience, looking back at the way we lived our life.

A recent study by the University of Wisconsin–Madison and Princeton University found that "the people who were purposefully engaged in life tended to have better levels of physical functioning." In summary, the article says, "While pleasurable experiences may lift your spirits, the ones that leave you with a sense of purpose and meaningful relationships may do even more: protect the body against ill health."[1]

"I've been having migraines and insomnia," Phyllis told her doctor. "I feel like something is missing, but I can't say exactly what it is. I mean, I love my family and we have all we need. I'm good at my job as a teacher. Frankly, I don't know what's wrong."

"Well," the doctor said, "obviously your stress level is high, and first we need to do something about the physical symptoms you're having. Let's do some testing to rule out any serious conditions. But, tell me—have you ever identified your purpose, the reason you're here? From what I've observed in thirty years of practice, people are generally happier and healthier, overall, when they have a sense of purpose. When our current life is at cross purposes with our deeper values, this causes inner conflict, and can lead to some of the symptoms you're having."[2]

After some serious reflection, Phyllis decided to take a painting class. As she sat in front of the easel with her paintbrush in hand, she began to feel a passion she had experienced as a child. Her art teacher was impressed by her creativity and encouraged her to continue to the next level. With her husband's support, Phyllis quit her teaching job to pursue painting and designing, and she's been healthier and happier ever since.

Living "on purpose" begins with some soul-searching and reflection; the result of that process could unlock a door to satisfaction you've never dared to imagine. Here are some suggestions for identifying your purpose:

1. List the ten things you care most about, and why; then reduce that list to the most important three. For example,

you might write: "I care about the declining health of the world." Your purpose will relate to this core value. It might read like this: "I am here to do what I can to reverse humanity's slide toward chronic illness and early death."

2. Reflect on your life's direction. Start by looking back, way back, to the things that really "lit your fire" as a child. Many people began their journey toward their current vocation at the age of eight to ten. Others may have had some special interests at one point, but as life has happened to them, they've lost touch with where they really wanted to go. Thankfully, it is never too late to change. So as part of this exercise, project yourself to the end of your life. Looking back to right now, what would you want to see between now and then to experience a sense of meaning and fulfillment? As soon as you can do so, you should move in that direction.

3. Your mission in life is the specific task or tasks that have been entrusted to you (and possibly to no one else). Your goals and even your short-term objectives are a part of this. Your mission can be expressed in a "mission statement," such as: "My mission is to help as many people as possible achieve and maintain optimal health."

However we discover our purpose in life, that knowledge is a great treasure, since it is one of the things that make human beings special in the whole scope of creation. The stronger our sense of "calling" (or vocation) becomes, the more effective we will be in living life on purpose. At the same time we too will benefit from the energy and intentionality that comes from knowing why we're here, where we're going, and what our mission in life is, not to mention the satisfaction that comes from fulfilling it.

30

Get a Good Night's Sleep

Two bears are in a cave. The papa bear is wide awake. The mama bear is dozing off. "I told you not to have coffee before winter," she says.

based on a Gary Larson cartoon

What's your "sleep number"? Four, six, eight, or even more . . . *hours* per night? Or maybe you'd prefer to sleep through the whole winter! While sleep needs vary by age, gender, and individual, researchers from the Division of Sleep Medicine in Boston studied 82,969 nurses and found "mortality risk was lowest among nurses reporting seven hours of sleep per night. After adjusting for age, smoking, alcohol, exercise, depression, snoring, obesity, and history of cancer and cardiovascular disease, sleeping less than six hours or more than seven hours remained associated with an increased risk of death."[1]

"Fatigue as a result of chronic sleep deficits is linked with poor work performance, driving accidents, relationship problems, and mood problems like anger and depression."[2] A 2005 poll by Sleep in America found that

nearly two-thirds of American drivers—60 percent—reported driving drowsy in 2004; 4 percent had an accident or near-accident because they were too tired, or they actually dozed off while driving. Some 100,000 car crashes per year [and 1,500 deaths annually] are attributed to drowsy driving. . . . Sleep deprived drivers are just as dangerous as drunk drivers, reports Dr. Kaplan from Mayo Clinic. In one study, people who drove after being awake for seventeen to nineteen hours performed worse than those who had a blood alcohol level of .05 percent.[3]

This is roughly the percentage achieved by drinking two typical drinks (containing a total of 20 grams of alcohol) in one hour, starting from sober. In other words, driving while drowsy is about as dangerous as driving while intoxicated.

If you experience chronic insomnia or chronic fatigue due to lack of sleep, consult your physician. These symptoms can indicate an underlying condition such as depression, bipolar disorder, or sleep apnea, for which treatments are available. This was true for a teacher named Mike, who wrote:

> When you are sitting in a classroom with thirty-two pairs of little eyes watching you, it is not good to fall asleep! But that was what I was doing: falling asleep at work, in front of the TV, on the couch, and when I was driving. I came home after work to take a nap, then slept in my reclining chair while the TV blared, and dragged off to bed at nine o'clock, barely able to open my eyes. On weekends, I could easily sleep until noon and then take a nap in the afternoon. Then, my dear wife complained that when I did go to bed, I snored like a hog. Life was basically miserable! Fortunately, my primary physician . . . referred me to an accredited sleep specialist. Sleep apnea was diagnosed and I began treatment. My wife didn't know what to do with me when I started getting up early on weekends. . . . I felt 100 percent better as the horrible tiredness slowly left me.[4]

Sleep is essential to good health because that's when our minds and bodies rest and rejuvenate themselves. Sleep has four stages, the lengths of which vary by person. At first you're in limbo between being awake and entering sleep. When you do finally fall asleep, your breathing remains regular, and your temperature goes down. The third and fourth stages are the deepest and most important, which is why frequently interrupted periods of sleep are not as effective. For about 25 percent of this time, your eyes rapidly move about as you dream (this is called REM sleep, for "rapid eye movement"). Your body is relaxed, energy is regained, and hormones are released for growth and development. Essentially, this is the time when your body relaxes, renovates, and repairs itself.

If you have trouble falling asleep or staying asleep, we suggest the following:

- Eat your last meal two to three hours before bedtime.
- Do not use caffeine or alcohol around bedtime.
- Make some improvements in your bedroom, such as room-darkening curtains or a more comfortable temperature at night.
- Use background noise (or "white noise") if your falling asleep is hindered by noise from outside your bedroom.
- Use earplugs if or when the situation requires it.
- If you exercise at night, give yourself a long enough break for your body to regain its sense of equilibrium.
- Try to go to bed around the same time each day, even on weekends.
- Read, listen to music, or "journal" for a half hour after you get into bed, as long as these activities help you relax.
- Include a hot bath in this routine if or when you are able to do so.
- Avoid activities close to bedtime that might make you uneasy or anxious, such as certain movies or the late news.
- Don't take your work to bed—for example, by taking your laptop along. Work or the Internet can take hours instead of minutes.
- Be sure that your bed, your bedding, and your pillows are all comfortable.

Sleep is one of God's gifts. It is meant to refresh and enrich us and renew our strength and vitality. Some people feel guilty about sleeping even seven or eight hours, because they measure their life by "productivity," whatever that means to them. But sound evidence exists that sleep is right up there in importance with proper diet and exercise for health and longevity.

31

Get and Keep Your Affairs in Order

Waiting for the fish to bite
or waiting for wind to fly a kite
or waiting around for Friday night
or waiting, perhaps, for their Uncle Jake
or a pot to boil, or a Better Break
or a string of pearls, or a pair of pants
or a wig with curls, or another chance.
Everyone is just waiting.

Dr. Seuss, *The Places You'll Go*

A 2007 poll found that although 76 percent of American adults say everyone needs a will, 57 percent do not have one. The most likely explanation is that most of us don't want to think about dying, and making a will forces us to do that. So we wait. Many wait too long.[1]

Few of us would take a trip without making elaborate plans about who will care for the dog, water the plants, and gather up the mail. One of the important lessons of any major disaster is that we never know when we might suddenly be out of time. If we do not have our affairs in order before time runs out, our loved ones will have to try to make sense of those affairs, and some court will decide who gets what.

Getting our affairs in order can bring a sense of peace and tranquility as we face an unknown future. Knowing that our cherished possessions and the people dear to us will be okay when we are no longer here can ease the mind like almost nothing else.

Seventy-eight-year-old Emma fell one day while walking to the corner store. She suffered a broken hip and was hospitalized for two weeks, followed by six weeks in a nursing home. Thankfully, her recovery was hastened by the fact that she truly had her affairs in order. Her grandson, who lived in a nearby town, knew where she kept all of her health and financial records. He brought her medical history file to the hospital, and soon all of Emma's medications and treatments were ordered to seamlessly transfer her medical needs to the hospital environment. Her bills were all paid on time and her friends were notified from a list she had prepared ahead of time. Even her little dog was immediately cared for as her neighbor came in and knew exactly where the food was kept and when the dog needed to be walked. Through her advance planning, Emma was freed to direct all her energies into getting well.

There are three main categories of concerns to put in order:

Personal Records: These include your full legal name, social security number, legal residence, date and place of birth, parentage and ancestry, names and addresses of spouse and children (location of death certificate if deceased), location of living will or other advance directive, location of birth certificate and certificate of marriage, divorce, and citizenship (passport, for example), list of employers and dates of employment, education and military records, religious affiliation, name of church, names of clergy, memberships in organizations and awards received, funeral and burial preferences (requests or prearrangements).

Financial Records: A list of insurance policies, bank accounts, real estate, and other valuables; sources of income and assets; Social Security and Medicare info; investment income (stocks, bonds, property, and brokers' names and addresses); insurance info (life, health, and property) with policy numbers and agents' names; bank account numbers (checking, savings, and credit unions); location of safe deposit boxes; copy of most recent income tax return; liabilities with details about how and when paid; location of mortgages and car titles; credit card and charge account names and numbers; property taxes; location of all personal valuables.

Legal Documents: This includes your will or trust, standard power of attorney or a durable power of attorney (to be used if a person is unable to make own decisions), and advance directive (describes your wishes about health care if you are not able to decide for yourself). Remember to specify if you desire anything to be taken out of your estate as a final gift to the work of your church or another favorite charity.[2]

Millions of people, indeed many famous or wealthy people, have died without a valid will, including presidents Abraham Lincoln, Andrew Johnson, and Ulysses S. Grant, as well as billionaire Howard Hughes and the painter Pablo Picasso. Don't allow your name to be added to that list.

32

Get Out There

I cannot endure to waste anything as precious as autumn sunshine by staying in the house. So I spend almost all the daylight
hours in the open air.

Nathaniel Hawthorne

How things have changed since Hawthorne's day, with much
of the change occurring within the past few years. In 2000, one
article reported that "67 percent of all Americans participate in
some sort of recreational activity at least once a month (defined
as anything from swimming to snowboarding), compared with
50 percent six years ago. Three in 10 Americans have enjoyed at
least six different recreational activities in the past year."[1]

However, by 2003 the Roper Report on Outdoor Recreation
in America (the most recently published such report) revealed
the following:

- There was a 5 point drop between 2001 and 2003 in the
  percentage of the public reporting participation in recreational activities several times per week (26% versus 21%)
  and a 7 point drop in those reporting participation several
  times per month (29% versus 22%).
- The drop in frequency of participation was especially noteworthy among young adults, a trend first noted in the 2001
  survey. It is noteworthy that this group reports high access
  to the Internet. 18- to 29-year-olds are now less likely to be
  frequent recreation participants (19%) than Americans between the ages of 30 and 44 (24%) or those 45 to 59 (22%).

- Four in 10 young adults are likely to engage in recreation either less than monthly or never.
- Previous surveys demonstrate widespread public recognition of the positive contributions to quality of life resulting from participation in outdoor recreation. The public links recreation to overall happiness, family unity, health, improved educational opportunities, and deterrence of crime and substance abuse. Declines in participation in so many recreational activities and the overall frequency of participation clearly put the benefits arising from recreation participation at risk.[2]

This trend away from participating in outdoor recreation, despite its perceived health benefits, parallels another trend, toward inactivity, especially among young people, and its inevitable result. "The prevalence of overweight in children ages 6–11 increased from 4.0 percent in 1971–74 to 17.5 percent in 1999–2004. The prevalence of overweight in adolescents ages 12–19 increased from 6.1 percent to 17.0 percent."[3]

The following statistics identify at least one cause:

- Number of minutes per week that the average child watches television: 1,680
- Percentage of day care centers that use TV during a typical day: 70
- Percentage of parents who would like to limit their children's TV watching: 73
- Percentage of 4- to 6-year-olds who, when asked to choose between watching TV and spending time with their fathers, preferred television: 54
- Hours per year the average American youth spends in school: 900 hours

- Hours per year the average American youth watches television: 1,500

It's not just the kids either. The same source said, "According to the A. C. Nielsen Co., the average American watches more than 4 hours of TV each day (28 hours/week, or 2 months of nonstop TV-watching per year). In a 65-year life, that person will have spent 9 years glued to the tube."[4]

Computers and computer games, the Internet, cell phones, PDAs, iPods, and just about anything electronic also contribute to the problem of physical inactivity, or even with the realization that one is inactive.

Anything that keeps you in your chair or glued to a screen is less healthy than actually moving around. So, if you think that limiting your TV time would be healthy, then apply the same principle to your computer or anything else that steals the time and energy you could be spending outdoors.

As you go, notice the little things, such as the beauty of a columbine or a hummingbird, as well as things that are simply majestic, like a mountain or the ocean. And let the Maker of the columbine and hummingbird and the mountains and the seas—and you!—speak to your soul.

33

Hang Loose or Stress Could Get You

> If you ask what is the single most important key to longevity, I would have to say it is avoiding worry, stress and tension. And if you didn't ask me, I'd still have to say it.
>
> George Burns

Chronic negative stress (distress) is one of the main killers of our modern age, even if it doesn't get the attention it deserves. In 1997, Bobbie and Jim published an article in the journal *Gastroenterology Nursing*, discussing how chronic distress can contribute to the development of (or aggravation of) many illnesses, including the following: asthma, cardiovascular disease, chronic fatigue syndrome, circulation problems in hands and feet, clinical depression, fibromyalgia, frequent colds, gastroesophageal reflux disease (GERD), hypertension (high blood pressure), irritable bowel syndrome, migraine headaches, stomach ulcers, stroke, and temporomandibular joint syndrome (TMJ).[1] In addition to all these conditions, here's one that isn't mentioned much—comfort eating—perhaps because "stressed" spelled backward is "desserts."

Dr. Hans Selye (1907–1982) was a Canadian endocrinologist of Austro-Hungarian origin who pioneered the study of stress and its impact on modern life. In fact, Selye originated the use of the word *stress* in this context, using the words *distress* for negative stress and *eustress* for good stress (stress that comes

113

from apparently good sources). One of his major points was that stress is pervasive in modern society and that in terms of the way the body responds to stress, it doesn't matter very much whether the source is negative or positive. What matters most is how you handle it—how you "adapt" to it or "cope" with it.

Selye wrote: "No one can live without experiencing some degree of stress all the time. You may think that only serious disease or intensive physical or mental injury can cause stress. This is false. Crossing a busy intersection, exposure to a draft, or even sheer joy are enough to activate the body's stress mechanism to some extent. Stress is not even necessarily bad for you; it is also the spice of life, for any emotion, any activity causes stress. But, of course, your system must be prepared to take it. The same stress which makes one person sick can be an invigorating experience for another."[2]

Joan was a regular "Energizer Bunny." Working in a high-stress job during the day, going to graduate school at night, and volunteering in various positions at her church, she really felt she was doing what God wanted her to do. "I held it all together until the stress became so great that I experienced major burnout. I had all the classic symptoms—perpetual exhaustion, insomnia, weight gain, irritability, depression, anxiety, plus a few panic attacks. Instead of enjoying what I was doing, I felt overwhelmed, and just wanted out. From this very frightening experience I learned to pace myself, to take time for fun and relaxation, to spend time with friends, and that I didn't have to do it all, or be involved in everything."

Since most of us cannot permanently withdraw to the mountains or monastery, the main issue is how we try to reduce our stress quotient, while learning to manage well our physical, emotional, sociological, and spiritual reactions to stressors that cannot be changed. Even if we did try to run from our stressors, new ones (from without or from within) would take their place.

Physically speaking, rest and relaxation (with some play thrown in, when possible) are essential to stress management. God rested when His creation work was finished, and then He sanctified that day of rest, both literally for the people of Israel and as a principle of life that is still valid in the Christian era. God valued rest so much He made it one of His Ten Commandments. As Spanish adventurer, author, and poet Miguel de Cervantes (1547–1616) said, "The bow cannot always stand bent, nor can human frailty subsist without some lawful recreation."

Psychologically, negative emotions including anxiety, anger, resentment, and an overall lack of serenity can all be related to stress that is not well managed. You may be familiar with these sayings: "Don't sweat the small stuff" and "It's all small stuff." From a faith perspective, it is possible to gain a different perspective of today's stressors by asking, "In the light of eternity, how important is this thing that has me so upset?"

Sociologically, as Selye said, relationships are often damaged by stress that is not well managed. People respond to pressure in unique ways, so it is possible for two people (including spouses) who are experiencing the same stressor to have entirely different reactions. One may be frantic; the other relaxed and confident. Such differences can kill a marriage—or strengthen it if both spouses accept the other's differences and see that they are stronger and more balanced together than either might be alone.

In terms of spiritual management of stress, science is showing that people of faith often handle stress better than others. One study showed that 84 percent of the fifty seniors studied used prayer rather than other alternative forms of treatment such as exercise or humor to relieve stress.[3]

Stress can kill you if you don't manage it well. Faith, friends, laughter, recreation (which we like to call "re-creation"), and relaxation can restore and maintain your health in the face of the multiple and inevitable stressors of life.

34

Have at Least One Close Friend

The only reward of virtue is virtue; the only way to have a friend is to be one.

Ralph Waldo Emerson

Having at least one friend is one of the marks of good mental health. Friendships are an important part of a healthy lifestyle. Friends not only bring joy into our lives but meet one of our basic needs, that of belonging. Good friends enhance our self-esteem and are a much-needed cushion as we travel through life's valleys. Friends double our happiness and cut our grief in half. No wonder those of us blessed with good friends have a better chance of living longer, healthier lives.

An Australian research team followed 1,500 Australians for ten years looking for connections between their social world and their longevity. They concluded, "A network of good friends is more likely than close family relationships to increase longevity in older people." Furthermore, people with large networks of good friends outlived those with the fewest friends by 22 percent. In addition, the positive effects continued throughout the ten years of the study regardless of negative life events such as the death of a spouse.[1] Other studies are in progress to confirm these results. Meanwhile, if you want to live long, have a friend and be a friend—the more the better.

Friends are not just acquaintances but positive companions on our life's journey—not *fair-weather* friends who only seek us out during the good times or times when they can gain from us. The best of both worlds is when family members are also friends! Some of us have the joy as we grow older of being surrounded by family who genuinely care for us and can be trusted confidants and encouragers. This is truly a gift and seems to be rarer as we speed into the twenty-first century.

Bobbie's grandmother, Idie, was such an inspiration. Not only was she close to her family of origin—caring for her parents in their old age—but she also maintained friendships with her seven brothers and sisters through the years. As children we used to love watching the sisters when they got together, laughing and talking about old times. Idie and her husband lived in the same house most of their adult lives, nurturing their many friendships through the years. They got together often with three other couples and even took the vacation of their lives together, visiting the Grand Canyon when all the men retired.

One by one, beginning with Bobbie's grandfather, they all passed away until Idie was the only one remaining. Even then, she consistently made new friends through her church and neighborhood, filling her days with activity and helping. She was famous for the fancy butter cookies she made each holiday for everyone from the postman to the grandchildren. Idie had a host of healthy relationships; she was connected and a joy to all who knew her until she passed away at age 94.

A study from Switzerland looking into the association between social relationships and survival of octogenarians came to interesting conclusions. The five-year study followed 295 people, looking at the effects of kinship and friendship networks. "Our analyses indicate that . . . the existence of close friends is a central component in the patterns of social relationships of oldest adults, and one which is significantly associated with survival. Overall, the protective effect of social relationships on survival is more related to the quality of those

117

relationships [close friends] than to the frequency of relation-ships [regular contacts]."[2]

Dr. Henry Cloud contends that lack of healthy relationships can lead to a wide range of addictions. "People are usually addicted to a specific substance, such as alcohol, cocaine, speed, or food. But people can also feel addicted to activi-ties, such as sex, gambling, work, destructive relationships, religiosity, achievement, and materialism. These substances and activities never satisfy, however, because they don't deal with the real problem. We don't really need alcohol, street drugs, or sex. We can live very well without these things. However, we really do need relationship, and we cannot live very well without it."[3]

Healthy friendships are vital to a joy-filled life. Having even one good friend who really cares is one of the keys to health and longevity. One of our favorite spiritual writers, Henri Nouwen, wrote, "The friend who can be silent with us in a moment of despair or confusion, who can stay with us in an hour of grief and bereavement, who can tolerate not knowing, not healing, not curing . . . this is a friend who cares."[4]

Before there were psychiatrists and counselors, there were friends who took long walks together, sharing their joys and their concerns, laughing or weeping together, depending on the circumstances each of them faced. In sharing life this way, they were fulfilling biblical descriptions of friendship, including that we are to bear one another's burdens, weep with those who weep, and rejoice with those who rejoice. Life can be lonely sometimes, and very, very hard. But in such times it is good to know we have both human friends and a supernatural Friend, who is described as a friend who sticks closer than a brother.

35

Hold On to Hope

Most of the important things in the world have been accomplished by people who have kept on trying when there seemed to be no hope at all.

Allan K. Chalmers

Dr. Viktor Frankl, a Jewish psychiatrist, survived a Nazi concentration camp to write *Man's Search for Meaning*, in which he describes the perspective he had to adopt if he wished to survive and help his fellows in despair gain new hope: "I was struggling to find the reason for my sufferings, my slow dying," Frankl wrote. "In a last violent protest against the hopelessness of imminent death, I sensed my spirit piercing through the enveloping gloom. I felt it transcend that hopeless, meaningless world, and from somewhere I heard a victorious 'Yes' in answer to my question of the existence of an ultimate purpose."[1]

Such stories of hope's victory over despair inspire us. We hear about people receiving financial help at the last minute, finding a job when they were about to lose everything, receiving life-saving medical care when needed, finding a lost brother, sister, or other family member or friend after many years of searching, a lost pet finding its way home again, someone who has moved through and beyond a tragic loss, someone whose diagnosis was grim but made a full recovery by clinging to hope.

In *The Anatomy of Hope*, hematologist/oncologist Dr. Jerome Groopman shares what he learned, primarily from his patients, in thirty years of practice. "Hope is the elevating feeling we experience when we see—in the mind's eye—a path to a better future. Hope acknowledges the significant obstacles and deep pitfalls along that path. True hope has no room for delusion. Clear-eyed, hope gives us the courage to confront our circumstances and the capacity to surmount them. For all my patients, hope, true hope, has proved as important as any medication I might prescribe or any procedure I might perform."[2]

It's not easy to have hope when life is falling down around us and we are in the middle of some of our darkest days. For most of us, there is the temptation to give in to despair, but those who have come through the "dark night of the soul" will tell you that hope was the thread that wove itself through their circumstances and kept them going. True hope is based on trust in a larger Reality than our own, that there is Someone bigger than we are Who is in control and Who knows the ultimate outcome of our lives. By faith we cling to that hope, which the New Testament describes as an anchor for the soul (see Heb. 6:19).

Hope and expectation are not the same. Jamie Shane, a staff writer for the Naples, Florida, *Daily News* writes:

> Isn't it funny how we fill our lives with expectations and then wander around wondering why we feel so unsatisfied? The creation of expectation is the ultimate form of self-sabotage, and it builds a strange stage for unhappiness. Creating expectation is a badly entrenched thought pattern, a gift from a culture that is perpetually looking ahead to better times regardless of how good the current times are. Some folks would call this good, old fashioned hope. Hope is not expectation. The difference between hope and expectation: hope is open, expectation is closed. Hope is a verse of "Que Sera, Sera." Expectation is a history lecture—no music at all and little room for interpretation. Hope is liberating and trusting. Expectation is the complete opposite.[3]

Hope and positive thinking also are not the same. Positive thinking is a psychological process used to combat pessimism. Research has shown that individuals who are hopeful and optimistic fare better in getting beyond their depression than those who are pessimistic and negative, and that being hopeful actually leads to a decrease in depression. Dr. Martin Seligman writes: "I've come to believe that low self-esteem, thinking you're worthless, is the least of all of these worries in depression. Once a depressed person becomes active and hopeful, self-esteem always improves. Bolstering self-esteem without changing hopelessness, without changing passivity, accomplishes nothing."[4]

"Hope" can be detrimental when it is based on fantasy or wishful thinking. This can be true of someone who has been diagnosed with a terminal illness and who still refuses to put his or her affairs in order, for example, or to try for reconciliation with estranged loved ones. "It is important in these cases for those caring for the patient not to offer them false hope of a cure or a miracle, but to redirect the patient to a new hope. This hope must be based on truth and not unrealistic expectations. Robert Frost said it well: 'Hope does not lie in a way out, but in a way through.'"[5]

Hope is a vital component of health and well-being. The result of hope is inner character, joy, steadfastness, perseverance, peace, serenity, and confidence. Hope is one of the strongest words of the Bible, occurring over one hundred times. It is planted in our hearts by God, in whose Word real hope trusts, for He will certainly bring to pass what He has promised, and He will never let go of us, even when, in our despair, we may be tempted to let go of Him.

36

Keep an Eye on Your Eyes

The eyes, like sentinels, hold the highest place in the body.

Cicero

We all treasure our eyes as our windows on the world. When our windows start to blur or become cluttered with little floaters or spots, or when one area of our vision seems fuzzy or darker than the rest, we worry. According to Miranda Hitti, "A recent survey of 1000 adults shows that nearly half—47 percent—worry more about losing their sight than about losing their memory and their ability to walk or hear!"[1]Fourteen million Americans are visually impaired. Elias Zerhouni, MD, director of the National Institutes of Health, said, "This is the first national survey on vision since the mid-1970s, and it confirms that uncorrected visual impairment is a major public health problem."[2]

Age-related macular degeneration (ARMD) can result in the loss of central vision; blurred vision; distorted vision; or colors appearing to fade. It is the number one cause of blindness in people over 60 and occurs when the retina's blood filter ceases to function and does not receive proper nutrients from the bloodstream. It can be partial or complete and causes heartache for millions of seniors worldwide.

Shelly was an active, bright, 75-year-old widow living in her home on the beautiful Oregon coast, with a breathtaking view of the majestic ocean and coastal rock formations. She savored each day as she watched the sun set over the Pacific. One day as she was ordering lunch in a restaurant she noticed the lines

122

on the menu were wavy and she was having trouble reading the words. Alarmed, she went to the eye doctor that very day and was stunned to learn that she had developed a condition called macular degeneration. Worse yet, she learned that one of the contributing causes may have been viewing so many sunsets without protective sunglasses. She began treatment, expecting to overcome this aggravation as she had others throughout her lifetime. She increased her intake of vegetables, wore sunglasses faithfully in bright sun and, as her doctor had cautioned, was careful to avoid secondhand smoke. The treatments did temporarily stem the progression of the disease, but one day two years later Shelly woke to find her vision far worse. This time, treatments did not help and the day soon came when Shelly had to leave the home she loved and move to a retirement village where she could get the twenty-four-hour care she now needed. She finds solace in her music and new friends and assures us she can still "see" her beautiful ocean view because it is permanently imprinted in her mind's eye.

With ARMD, prevention beats prescription, hands down. The prescription for prevention is fairly simple: eat plenty of yellow and green vegetables every day (spinach, kale, turnip greens, collards, mustard greens, squash, green peas, broccoli, pumpkin, and corn). These foods contain rich nutrients such as lutein and zeaxanthin. Eggs are a good source as well. Whole food concentrates that contain foods high in these nutrients are also good preventative medicine.[3]

A pilot study done at the DVA Medical Hospital of North Chicago indicates that lutein may improve vision. Researchers demonstrated short-term positive effects in visual function after patients incorporated more lutein into their diets. Fourteen male patients between ages 61 and 79 with early symptoms of ARMD such as blurred vision or loss of central vision ate four to seven servings of spinach weekly. Researchers saw improvements ranging from 60 to 92 percent on several visual function tests in all patients.[4] The equivalent of one cup of raw spinach daily is all it takes. To augment this natural treatment regimen, you might consider taking a daily multivitamin containing lutein.

Cataracts are caused by proteins in the eye binding to each other, causing a cloudy spot to form on the lens of the eye. This causes a host of hassles such as poor nighttime vision, halos around lights, and sensitivity to glare. Cataracts are slow-growing and need to "ripen" before surgery can be done to replace the lens.

Glaucoma is characterized by increased pressure in the eye that can cause blindness. It can come on suddenly or slowly, and the symptoms we need to watch for are blind spots, loss of vision, or poor night vision. Glaucoma can be successfully treated with prescription eyedrops, but it is a condition for which there is no cure. This is one important reason to see your ophthalmologist yearly for a thorough eye exam.

Vision impairment is linked to longevity because it affects our quality of life so drastically. Falls and accidents are much more common in those with vision impairment, which can lead to serious problems and decreased quality of life and mental health. Studies show that impaired vision can bring on or worsen depression. Formerly active people do not feel as secure if vision begins to change. Loss of vision can erode our independence and steal our treasured pastimes along with the health benefits that come from mobility and interaction with friends and family.

Modern science has given us many treatments to help retain and restore eyesight, but we trust that you will become proactive about preserving your windows on the world and embrace prevention as the key to maintaining healthy vision. Even if you don't like spinach or broccoli or kale or the other vegetables high in lutein, project yourself to age 70 and beyond as a blind or vision-impaired person. Looking back, the alternative of saving your vision by changing your diet now might make some lutein-rich vegetables every day a lot more palatable, don't you think?

37

Keep Your Heart Smart

The best six doctors anywhere
And no one can deny it
Are sunshine, water, rest, and air,
Exercise and diet.
These six will gladly you attend
If only you are willing
Your mind they'll ease
Your will they'll mend
And charge you not one shilling.[1]

Anonymous

Heart health is at the forefront of the war on aging in America, and with good reason—heart disease continues to be the number one killer nationwide. But does anyone know whether heart disease is caused by poor genes or poor choices? The answer—definitely *both*. You can't change your family tree, but if you have a family history of heart disease and want to improve your own odds, you can actually do so if you take the threat seriously enough.

Recent studies show that lifestyle carries more weight for prevention than genetics. Carl Eisdorfer, MD, director of the University of Miami Center on Aging, states: "The best data shows that only about one-third of longevity is due to genes. The most important factors are behavioral: eating too much, eating the wrong foods, alcohol, and drugs, how you view stress, how you deal with it—whether you are connected to family, if you have an extended family."[2]

Sometimes the data is very focused, as when researchers from the Harvard School of Public Health found that eating one to two servings of fish a week reduces death from heart disease by 36 percent.[3] Even being happy instead of depressed can be heart-healthy. A Swedish study reported that people diagnosed with depression are 1.5 times more likely to develop coronary heart disease.[4] A report in the journal *Heart* showed a 50 percent increase in blood flow to the heart while watching happy versus sad movies. Watching a comedy boosted blood flow to a level equal to that of doing aerobic exercise or taking a cholesterol-lowering statin, the report stated.[5]

Stan's dad had his first heart attack at age 45 and died several years later when Stan was still in medical school. It was a sobering time and Stan vowed to adopt a healthy lifestyle. He decided that taking up running would solve the problem and regularly got up at 5:00 a.m. to run for thirty to forty-five minutes before hospital rounds. He continued this regimen for the next twenty years, believing it would prevent heart disease. A heart scan proved otherwise; Stan's doctor said, "Your scan shows a high calcium score, indicating accumulation of plaque in your arteries." Stan left the clinic, shaken and disbelieving, forcing himself to carefully mull over the doctor's words. He knew that the high calcium score, combined with out-of-balance cholesterol, was an ominous sign.

With mortality staring him in the face and all his hopes and dreams for the future suddenly at risk, Stan and his wife, Joan, prayed for wisdom and guidance. Motivated by the latest research and with the help of his doctor, Stan devised a lifestyle plan to stabilize and hopefully even reverse the plaque buildup. He and Joan evaluated overall stressors as well as diet and exercise and immediately put changes into effect. They asked for prayer and support from friends and family, adjusted work schedules, and increased exercise to an hour of cardio four to five days a week, with some outdoor activity on weekends. They selected Dr. Ornish's reversal diet as the meal plan, and Joan adopted a whole new way of cooking and preparing meals, with only a small percentage of calories coming from fat each day.

The research is clear that certain kinds of foods and exercise are vital to winning over heart disease. You don't have to become a marathon runner; walking, biking, or swimming are good alternatives. You don't have to eat only bean sprouts. But you do need to pay attention to the proven basics. Numerous excellent meal plans are available that you can tailor to your specific situation with the advice of your doctor. But you don't need a doctor to tell you that. All the experts recommend eating at least ten servings of fruits and veggies a day! This may seem like an overwhelming assignment at first, but you can improve, especially when you incorporate supplements such as whole food concentrates into your daily diet.[6]

While you may think it hard to accomplish your goals in this area, if you could project yourself to the end of your life, what would you give for an extra five years, three years, or even one year? Heart disease could easily rob you of that much time, if not more. With that in mind, when is the best time to begin turning back that clock?

You can begin to make healthy choices, day by day, and all of these can affect your heart health long-term. Yes, change is hard and you may get discouraged, even when you know what must be done. Depression, overwork, substance abuse, lack of preventative medical advice, and lack of support from family and friends can all contribute to failure, even when we want to change. But family and friends can also contribute to our success when we make it clear that keeping our ticker ticking is something we want to facilitate, because we want to have as much time as possible to enjoy living—with them.

So make those hard choices and changes and then enlist the help and support of others. Once you have your support network in place, do everything you can to adopt a lifestyle that will help you thrive and have a happy heart!

38

Keep Your Mind Sharp

When I was young I couldn't remember anything, whether it had happened or not.

Mark Twain

Our memories are among our most treasured possessions. We fondly remember the best of times, while trying to forget the worst of times.

You've probably been in a situation where you experienced an embarrassing lapse of memory, say, at a social or business gathering, and you're a little nervous. As a result, you block on your best friend's name, as in, "John, I want you to meet my old friend _____."

As we age, we may struggle to remember some things, but most seniors do not have enough loss of memory to prevent them from living a normal life. However, Dr. William Cheshire

Jr. from the Mayo Clinic, writes, "For many people, the prospect of deterioration in brain function is feared more than any other ailment of aging. Joints may give way and vision dim without eroding personal integrity. The brain, however, is essential to who we are. Its grey matter is the centerpiece of the living tapestry of personal identity."[1]

Keeping your mind sharp with the passing years can be a challenge. You may find it harder to learn new things or to remember vocabulary words and familiar names on the spot. Although your long-term memory may be intact and even more vivid than your recall of things that happened just a few years ago, retrieval of those earlier memories slows down, like a computer whose RAM is almost maxed out. In addition, your ability to concentrate on more than one thing at a time may be affected.

At the outset of a three-year study of 498 elderly people by the Johns Hopkins School of Medicine, 16 were found to have normal cognitive function, 133 had mild cognitive difficulties, and 349 had dementia (severe problems with reasoning and memory.) During the period of the study, 136 of the participants died, only one of whom had demonstrated normal cognitive function at the start. Of the rest who died, 24 had demonstrated mild impairment and 111 had demonstrated dementia. The authors of the study called for more research to find ways to prevent this devastating impact of disordered memory and reasoning on the survival of elderly persons.[2]

June was a high-level executive secretary and enjoyed keeping up with her many responsibilities. She could make plane reservations in an instant, while balancing the day's receipts and greeting clients by name as they walked through the door. At home she easily coordinated all the family get-togethers, kept up with her six grandchildren's activities, and remembered everyone's birthday! But as she turned 62, June began to notice some lapses. Sometimes she stopped mid-sentence as she tried to find the word she was looking for. She was having difficulty remembering the time of her favorite TV program or the phone number of a business associate she had previously called often. Too worried to go to the doctor, she kept her fears to herself until one day her daughter brought up her concern. "Mom," she tentatively began, "you know how much I care about you and want you to be happy and healthy. I've noticed that you seem to be forgetting things more often, and sometimes even seem at a loss for words. Are you okay?"

Her daughter's love and concern motivated June to see her doctor. Several weeks later, during a follow-up appointment, the doctor carefully explained that June was showing early signs of dementia. She was terrified at first by this diagnosis, but with the loving support of her family she faced her challenges with courage, and with the help of new medication experienced some reduction of her symptoms.

As we age, we fear that our cognitive powers will slowly depart. Thankfully, there are steps we can take to slow down or prevent memory problems, or even to fight off the dreaded Alzheimer's disease.[3]

The following suggestions are all supported by medical research:

- Don't "jar" your brain. Wear a helmet when biking or skiing, make sure your home is free of hazards that could cause falls, and always wear a seat belt when in or on a moving vehicle.
- Maintain vital relationships with family or multiple friends.
- Exercise your brain by doing puzzles and games.
- Learn a new skill, hobby, or language, or learn to play a musical instrument. Visit a museum, read more, write

letters, or keep a diary. For a real challenge, try writing in the diary with your non-dominant hand.

- Exercise regularly. This improves the blood flow to your brain.
- Get your nutrition from whole foods. Recent studies are focusing on oxidative stress as a primary cause of Alzheimer's.
- Make lists of things you need to remember.
- Use associations as memory aids—such as mental pictures for names (Mr. Carpenter, Mrs. Baker, Mr. Green).

If you do these things, you'll be less likely to be in this situation: "John, I want you to meet my wife, _____. Honey, tell him your name."

39

Keep Your "Wow" Working

Sophistication scares the wonder out of us. Cynicism downright annihilates it. Wonder leaves no room for meanness, for where wonder is, kindness is also. Wonder isn't harsh, but as gentle as rain.

Connie Powers

Once there was a little girl who was home with her father during a terrible lightning storm. At one point the father realized his daughter was up in the attic by herself and he was concerned that she might be afraid. When he got up to her, he found her with her nose plastered to the window. He asked her if she was afraid and she replied, "No, Daddy. God is taking my picture."

Oh, the wonders of childhood! Close your eyes and think back to a time when you were a child and were experiencing something so exciting, mysterious, and surprising that it filled you with a sense of wonder, awe, and amazement. It was so real that you could see it, feel it, hear it, smell it, and taste it all at the same time. Childhood wonder is like that.

However, by the time we reach middle age, we've experienced many "watersheds in our lives when our dreams die, when our imaginations become hardened along with our arteries and wonder goes fleeting out the windows."[1] Watersheds that diminish our sense of wonder can include any adultish thing, such as being too busy, holding a job, raising a family, or experiencing times of trauma and loss. Negative emotions such as anger, worry, stress, anxiety, and depression also drain our wonder reservoir. One symptom is how often we can pass a field of wild irises, or even a single columbine, without stopping long enough to let our "wow" work and our appreciation for their Maker gush forth.

"The late '60s folk legends Peter, Paul, and Mary . . . had a song called, 'Puff the Magic Dragon.' It was, of course, a song about the fantasy worlds of children and the loss of innocence . . . [for] one day the scales of wonder fall like rain. We cease hearing the voice of childhood, and even the voice of God, because our *lives* become louder. The crescendo of our possessions, the noise of our careers, the soul-smothering volume of everyday existence drowns out that still small voice that comes with the breath of a light whisper."[2]

Losing our sense of wonder can dull our creativity, diminish our sense of purpose and joy, and even steal our passion for life, leaving us disenchanted, disillusioned, and dissatisfied—with life in general and the things and people around us.

Albert Einstein said, "He who can no longer pause to wonder and stand rapt in awe, is as good as dead: his eyes are closed." Without doubt, then, retaining or regaining a childlike sense of wonder, awe, and passion for life is the way to experience life to the full, versus dying a little bit, day by day. Not only so, if you have children, your wow-ability is going to be contagious. "If a child is to keep alive his inborn sense of wonder," writes Rachel Carlson, "he needs the companionship of at least one adult who can share it, rediscovering with him the joy, excitement and mystery of the world we live in."[3]

For some adults, "wow" is a central component of their personality, affecting their life in many ways, perhaps most significantly their ability to savor even the small things that other "grown-ups" just take for granted. This quality is rare, however. In fact, I (Dave) have known only one adult who lives this way consistently. Whether he's observing a wildflower poking through the snow, a particular rock formation, or the golden splendor of a single aspen leaf in the fall, Monte Swan comes closest to my own understanding of what Jesus may have meant when he spoke of adults becoming "as little children" so they can see the kingdom of heaven. In the book I helped Monte write, *Romancing Your Child's Heart*, we give many practical suggestions about how to renew your sense of wonder and share it with your children, if you still have some at home. If you're a grandparent, rediscovering your sense of wonder with your grandchildren could help you live a longer and happier life. For example:

A spontaneous expression of genuine wonder and curiosity excites a child's interest and points inevitably to God in a way that woos rather than repels a young mind. "Wow! Look at that hummingbird!"—as it dive-bombs your heads—"I wonder how it can fly like that—up, down, sideways, any which way it wants. I wonder if it can fly upside down?"

These comments may lead you to read descriptions in guide-books or to visit websites . . . where you can learn any number of things about the seventeen species in North America, or the three hundred and twenty species worldwide, of the bird family Trochilidae. For now, however, the "Wow!" will suffice.[4]

Sir Isaac Newton wrote, "I do not know what I may appear to the world; but to myself I seem to have been only like a boy playing on the seashore, and diverting myself in now and then finding a smoother pebble or a prettier shell than ordinary, whilst the great ocean of truth lay all undiscovered before me."[5]

40

Know the Skinny on Fat

The older you get, the tougher it is to lose weight because by then, your body and your fat are really good friends.

Anonymous

When we were growing up, the skinny on fat was much simpler. Fat was fat and that was that. Most of us ate it without a second thought. We drank whole milk with cream floating on the top, consumed cheeseburgers, bacon, and french fries with gusto, grilled nicely marbled steaks, and even fried with Crisco, which was made from partially hydrogenated cottonseed oil, one of the first "trans fats."

Toward the end of the twentieth century fat got a bad name. "Fat is bad," we heard. "Low fat is better." Unfounded claims were made that low-fat was even healthier. An entire food industry was developed to produce low-fat foods, some of them higher in calories than similar products high in fat.

Today we're bombarded with information about fat. There's saturated fat; monounsaturated fat; polyunsaturated fat; omega-3; -6, and -9 fatty acids; and trans fat. Some fats are good for you. Some are harmful. But you don't have to be a scientist to know which is which, because in general, most healthy fats come from natural sources; most man-made fats are less healthy. In terms of natural fats, unsaturated fats are healthier than saturated fats. Omega-3 and -6 fatty acids are essential to health and must be obtained through one's diet.

The names for the various fats describe their chemical composition. Saturated fats are "saturated" with hydrogen atoms. Butter, clarified butter, suet, tallow, lard, coconut, cottonseed and palm kernel oils, dairy products (especially cream and cheese), and some meats are high in saturated fat.

Your body needs fat because it is an energy source and a nutrient used in the production of such important things as cell membranes and compounds that help regulate heart rate, blood pressure, blood clotting, your nervous system, and blood vessel constriction. Fat also carries vitamins A, D, E, and K from your food into your body. Fat helps maintain healthy hair and skin, protects your vital organs, and insulates your body.

Hydrogenated and partially hydrogenated oils are called "trans fats." Hydrogenation solidifies vegetable oil so that it resembles real food. Vegetable oil is "hydrogenated" under pressure with hydrogen gas at 250 to 400 degrees Fahrenheit for several hours—in the presence of a catalyst such as nickel or platinum. The name trans fat describes the new configuration of hydrogen atoms, which increases shelf life and makes the fat spreadable. For example, you can't spread pure corn oil on your toast, but you can spread margarine containing hydrogenated corn oil on your toast, a practice that at one time was heralded as healthier than using butter.

> According to the National Academy of Sciences Institute of Medicine, there are "no known health benefits" associated with trans fats. In April 2006, the Harvard School of Medicine published the study "Trans Fatty Acids and Cardiovascular Disease" which showed that the elimination of industrially produced trans fats would prevent between 72,000 and 228,000 heart attacks each year, accounting for 6–19% of all annual heart attacks. Also, trans fats were associated with a "tripling of the risk of sudden death from cardiac causes."[1]

We see the heartbreak of obesity all around us. All we have to do is go to the local "all you can eat" buffet and observe the girth of some of the patrons. The popular TV show *The Biggest Loser* documents the struggle so well. It's not just how much we weigh but how much body fat we carry—usually all too visible around the middle in men, and in back in women. This is the dangerous visceral fat that collects in our abdominal cavity, crowding our vital organs and causing serious health problems.

So join the fight against fat and celebrate the new you. When you do, you'll follow the lead of former Arkansas Governor Mike Huckabee. In eighteen months time he "whittled 110 pounds from his 5-foot-11 frame, going from 280 pounds to a trim 170 pounds." Huckabee didn't plan on being an icon in the war against obesity. He simply wanted to get healthy after being diagnosed with type 2 diabetes. "Frankly," he said, "I was facing the fact that I was in the last decade of my life." It was a turning point for Huckabee, then just 48. He is quick to point out that the path he took involved commitment and hard work. He says he was a chronic overeater who hated to exercise. Huckabee warns, "There will never come a day where you can say, 'Wow!

I can wipe my brow and call it quits and go back to my ways because I have done this thing.'"[2]

Once fat cells are produced, they tend to stay with us our whole lives, demanding to be fed. This is why it is so hard for people who became overweight during childhood to shed the extra pounds and keep them off.[3] Perhaps you're one adult who understands this because it is the story of your life thus far. If so, and you have influence on the next generation, give them the skinny on fat, and do whatever is necessary to support any decision they make to change their eating habits.

41

Laugh More

Laughter is inner jogging.

Norman Cousins

Want to live longer? Laugh more. Laughter has multiple health benefits, and all it takes is a good joke, like, Guest: "Why does your dog sit there and watch me eat?" Hotel host: "I can't imagine, unless it's because you have the plate he usually eats from."

Or: Two antennae meet on a roof, fall in love, and get married. The ceremony isn't much, but the reception is excellent.

Are you laughing yet?

If yes, then your face is convulsing involuntarily. Your facial muscles, particularly your lips, are stretching and you have a peculiar expression in your eyes. Your vocal organs vibrate and then you utter a sequence of rhythmic expiratory sounds. You sound like you're choking as you gasp for breath, while your shoulders jerk and your entire body twists and shakes. If they didn't know you were laughing, observers might think you were having a seizure. But since you are laughing, they will most likely start laughing with you. It's just one of those things that humans do.

In one of the first studies linking humor appreciation with longevity, the researchers found that "adults who scored in the top one-quarter for humor appreciation were 35 percent more likely to be alive [seven years later] than those in the bottom quarter."[1]

From ancient times we have believed that laughter is good for us. The Greek poet Pindar said, "The best of healers is good cheer." Humor affects our bodies in major ways: biologically, psychologically, sociologically, and spiritually. We all can benefit from generating mirth wherever we go.

The physical and psychological responses to laughter have been studied the most. Laughter boosts the immune system, decreases stress hormones, lowers blood pressure, increases muscle flexion, exercises muscles (abdominal, facial, and respiratory) increases blood oxygenation, decreases pain, increases healing after surgery, promotes well-being, conditions the heart, and benefits lung disease.[2]

To reap the most benefit, your laughter usually has to be hearty and out loud. Most adult Americans laugh about fifteen times a day, while babies laugh hundreds of times a day. Humorist Larry Wilde insists, "A robust rib-rattler improves not only your mood but also your health. The physical act of laughing helps you stay alert, makes it easier to cope and lets you maintain your sanity when the world goes a little crazy."[3]

We see a sense of humor all through Scripture and know that our ability to laugh was orchestrated by God Himself. In fact the Bible teaches us that "a cheerful heart has a continual feast," and "a merry heart doeth good like a medicine."[4]

Laughter is a gift given at birth and if cultivated can smooth many a road bump all through life. Many parents love to recall the first time they heard their babies laugh. They videotape the day the occasional little chuckle gives way to a belly laugh and send it around the world. Babies see humor that often escapes us. The first time Jim and Bobbie's granddaughter dissolved into laughter at about four months of age was at the sight of her puppy racing and jumping through the piles of fall leaves. She quickly infected the whole family with her mirth.

Most children have a great sense of humor. And as Art Linkletter showed us so well, they say and do the funniest things! In the Dill family a comment by their oldest son has gone down in their history. At age four he was listening to a conversation about Bobbie's brother starting night school in the fall. He turned to us with huge, saucer eyes and asked, "Uncle George is gonna be a knight?" As a natural-born comic, he enjoyed the merriment and chance to make everyone laugh.

Some people have a special gift of spreading mirth. Robin Williams comes immediately to mind in his great movie *Patch Adams*. In fact, the Humor Foundation was established in Australia as a result of the work of Patch Adams. Actual Clown Doctor Units have been established in several major hospitals there.[5]

In the United States, a plastic surgeon at the University of Arkansas for Medical Sciences, Julio Hochberg, MD, brings a smile to his patients' faces with the help of three custom-made puppets named Dr. Hamburger, Nurse Fry, and Dr. Baby. Hochberg's patients at Arkansas Children's Hospital look forward to his Friday clinic, which features the puppets plus lots of laughs.[6]

Many of us have a family comic in our midst. Everyone loves Bobbie's sister, Peggy. She goes through life spreading a wave of humor. Her patients love her, and in the kidney dialysis unit where she works they line up to request her as their nurse. She sees the funny side of life and has a way of telling stories that transform your day! She just naturally lightens up everyone's mood as she travels through life.

So take advice from Larry Wilde: "Humor is nature's antidote for tension. Let it be your secret weapon when you're up to your eyeballs in alligators. It's fast, it's fun, it's free. No other stress buster can make this claim!"[7]

42

Lighten Up

Remember that fear always lurks behind perfectionism. Confronting your fears and allowing yourself the right to be human can, paradoxically, make you a far happier and more productive person.

Dr. David M. Burns

Some of us become perfectionists all by ourselves. In most cases we learn this perspective from parents or other adult mentors who usually only want the best for us. But they are not as aware as they could be of the degree to which they have tied their own self-esteem or personal hopes and dreams to our "success." For example, a parent who never finished college may push a gifted child to excel academically so he or she will have the best possible opportunity for advanced education, including training in one of the more lucrative professions.

Multiple studies have shown links between illness (mental or physical) and perfectionism. A May 2007 WebMD article by Miranda Hitti reviewed recent Swiss research that studied fifty men (average 42 years of age), twenty-four of whom scored high in perfectionism about personal standards and concern over mistakes. These men tended to be more anxious, neurotic, and exhausted than the others. When subjected to a stress-inducing test, the perfectionists had higher levels of cortisol,[1] which remained true for an hour after the test was over.[2]

When children are never able to measure up to the demands or expectations of those they really wish to please, they are likely to have some or all of the following attitudes:

- Fear, including fear of disapproval, making mistakes, or "failure"
- Inadequacy, inferiority, or guilt because nothing is ever quite good enough
- A black-and-white/all-or-nothing perspective—on the world in general—and the rigidity and intolerance that comes with it
- A sense of frustration that others can seem to be satisfied with their own work, while they cannot be satisfied with less than perfection, which remains unreachable; the result is often depression or other forms of mental illness, including obsessive-compulsive disorder
- Procrastination, possibly related to fear of failure and another reason to feel inadequate
- Resentment—though it may take years to become a conscious feeling—toward the people who pressured them to achieve not just excellence, but perfection

Many perfectionists excel in their field, while struggling in silence with the attitudes listed, the relational damage that results, and sometimes with the emotional baggage too. We believe it is possible that many sincere Christian parents place higher expectations on their children than is healthy. One of our friends, a doctor who wishes to remain anonymous, wrote about this in an article she called "The Dance," excerpted here with her permission:[3]

> Once upon a time there was a little girl whose parents were convinced was the smartest, most beautiful, most athletic, most interpersonally gifted, most bound-to-be-successful child who had ever been born. And they told her so. They wanted to be sure that she reached her full potential, so when she didn't act right, or when she got ideas about things that weren't in her best interest, they were careful to set her straight and make sure that she continued down the right path. . . .
>
> Sometimes the little girl wondered: *What if all of a sudden, I wasn't the smartest, most beautiful, most athletic, most interpersonally gifted, most bound-to-be-successful child who has ever been born. Who would I be? And what would my parents think about me?* Afraid of the answer, she began to dance as fast as she could to keep up the front.
>
> The little girl grew up and became a doctor . . . always dancing. She married and had two wonderful children of her own. And she kept dancing . . . until one day she felt very, very tired. Her legs slowed their pace, and finally they stopped. She couldn't dance any more. So she fell. It was a free-fall . . . down, down, down . . . until she thought she would suffocate if she fell any further. And as she fell, she kept telling her legs, "Get me back to the dancing place. Save me from this fall. What about the honor, the glory, the approval? I must keep dancing."
>
> But her legs wouldn't cooperate. She cursed her legs and told them they were bad. Then she cursed herself and told herself she was bad. And then she cursed everyone around her, whose fault the whole thing must have been in the first place. And she told them they were bad. All the while, she kept falling,

convinced that she would fall forever, and nothing she could do would make it stop.

So she cried. She cried as she had never cried before, sobbing from the pain and weariness of dancing all day and night for thirty years, even when she hadn't wanted to. She cried because she was letting down so many people. And once she started crying, she couldn't stop crying, either. . . . Until she cried to God. "I can't dance anymore. There's absolutely nothing left. I'm sorry. I have let You down." And even as she spoke those words, she suddenly stopped falling, with a jolt. She had been caught, and now was being held, even cradled by a hand that rocked her and gave her rest. And a voice said, "I never asked you to do that dance. I love you whether you can dance or not. I made you just the way you are—a reasonably intelligent, completely un-athletic, moderately interpersonally gifted child who isn't better than anyone else, but who is created so uniquely that no one can replace her. I don't want you to dance anymore. I want you to rest. I want you to sleep in My rocking hand and feel how much I love you. And then . . . ONLY THEN . . . I want you to go back up to land and let other people see what your life looks like when you're dancing for Me, and not for them."

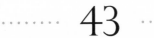

43

Live in the Now

Yesterday is history. Tomorrow is a mystery. And today? Today is a gift. That's why we call it the present.

Babatunde Olatunji

Every second of the day, life hurries past us at an alarming rate. The older we become, the faster it seems to go. We are great at fooling ourselves about life slowing down sometime in the future. It just isn't going to happen unless we do something to make it happen. As the movie character Ferris Bueller says, "Life moves pretty fast. If you don't stop and look around once in a while, you could miss it."[1]

People who are anxious or depressed often live the greater part of each day thinking about the past or worrying about the future. "Logically it does not make sense to worry about the future, as we don't ever live in the future. We live only in the present. Most of the things we fear don't happen anyway," says Christina Diaz. "Besides the main practical problem that exists with fearing the future is that you think about the future situation from the thoughts, emotions, and beliefs that you have NOW, which will be different when the future situation comes about. The living-ness is right now. Why waste time with something that hasn't happened when you can be with what is—totally?"[2]

Jesus said it best: "Therefore do not worry about tomorrow, for tomorrow will worry about itself. Each day has enough trouble of its own" (Matt. 6:34).

Does this mean it's wrong to plan for our future? Not at all. Not to plan in certain areas such as health, finances, career, retirement, and caring for your family is foolishness. The idea is to plan and then let it go, trusting that you have done what you've needed to do to take care of yourself and those you love.

Ever tell yourself that you will start that diet tomorrow, go back to school tomorrow, leave the job you hate *tomorrow*? This is living in the future. It's easy to imagine a better life, a thinner you, a job you love, the perfect mate, and on and on. But that vision will always remain a figment of your imagination unless you take steps *today* to make it happen. The result of living this way is anxiety and unhappiness, because you live life in a state of discontent, without peace or happiness. If you want a better future, set realistic and achievable goals today and move forward to make it happen. Mañana never comes.

Equally unhealthy is living in the past, full of regrets for what you did or didn't do, all those mistakes you made, people you hurt, people who hurt you. Rehashing the past locks you into living there, since your mind can really only focus on one thing at a time, and when it's focused on the past, enjoying today— much less actually experiencing it with all your senses—is nearly impossible. Once you decide to accept that you can't change the past, you can release it and your emotional attachment to it and live now.

Michael McGrath describes the following steps if you want to release your past: "The first step is to accept that it happened, no matter how traumatic or distasteful the experience was. After acceptance you can enter a state of peace when you realize that the past, all of it, good and bad experiences alike have helped to form and mold the person you are today. Next, realize that the past has some powerful lessons to teach you. Look for the positive learning experience that the past has taught you—use it as a learning tool. Make up your mind not to repeat those same mistakes, but to do things differently next time. And, finally, never use your past as an excuse to stay where you are, staying stuck. All you have is this moment and that is all you need to make changes."[3]

Tragic circumstances have a way of forcing us to live in the present. Tony Dungy, coach of the Indianapolis Colts, found this to be true after the suicide of his oldest son, James, in 2005. "It's probably something I won't come to grips with," Dungy says of his son's death. "But what it forces you to do is live in the present. It's hard to do, but that's what you have to do. You have to program yourself to live in the present. Make the present as good as you can make it, because you can't count on the future, and you can't go back and redo the past."[4]

Make up your mind to stop and smell the roses . . . today. After all, it's all you have. In the inimitable words of Henry David Thoreau, "You must live in the present, launch yourself on every wave, find your eternity in each moment. Fools stand on their island opportunities and look toward another land. There is no other land, there is no other life but this."[5]

44

Love and Be Loved

If you have love in your life, it can make up for a great many things you lack. If you don't have it, no matter what else there is, it's not enough.[1]

Ann Landers

One of the most beautiful descriptions of love was penned by the apostle Paul: "Love is patient, love is kind. It does not envy, it does not boast, it is not proud. It is not rude, it is not self-seeking, it is not easily angered, it keeps no record of wrongs. Love does not delight in evil but rejoices with the truth. It always protects, always trusts, always hopes, always perseveres. Love never fails" (1 Cor. 13:4–8).

Love in its purest form, then, is *more* than just a feeling. It is directed toward others, unselfishly. It often goes against what we would naturally do, and can require great sacrifice. As Jesus said, "Greater love has no one than this, that he lay down his life for his friends" (John 15:13).

Love is easy when people are easy to love. But what about loving the "unlovable," those people who seem to have few attractive qualities, or who appear to have little inner or outer beauty? In the tale "Beauty and the Beast," Belle, a beautiful young girl, is obligated to live at the home of the Beast in exchange for her father's freedom. Because the Beast is kind to her, her heart eventually turns toward him in love. At one point in the story Belle is allowed to visit her family, with the promise that she will return exactly one week later. When her return is delayed by her jealous sisters, the Beast's heart is broken. Belle finds him in the rose garden, dying. But when she says she loves him and weeps over him, her tears turn him into a handsome prince, releasing him from the spell that had made him a beast.

Redemptive love loves the unlovely—those who are hard to love or perhaps don't even seem to want or appreciate love. Of course our love can't transform "beasts" into "beauties." Only God knows the hidden beauty lying dormant in that unlovely or hard-to-love person, which just might surface when we love them.

Loving and being loved are just plain good for your health. Scientists have long known that happily married people live longer, have fewer heart problems and lower cancer rates, and enjoy other physical, mental, and social benefits as well.

- "According to one Harvard University study, married women are 20 percent less likely than single women to die of a variety of causes, including heart disease, suicide, and cirrhosis of the liver. Married men enjoy an even greater benefit—they're two to three times less likely to die of such causes than are single men."[2]
- "Dean Ornish, MD, compiled a number of studies on love and health in his book, *Love and Survival: The Scientific Basis for the Healing Power of Intimacy* (HarperCollins,

1998). He described one study of nearly ten thousand married men with no previous history of angina (chest pains). Despite high risk factors such as high cholesterol, high blood pressure, and diabetes, men who felt loved by their wives experienced half the angina as men who felt their wives did not show them love."[3]

- "Levels of the 'anti-aging' hormone DHEA, which produces feelings of youth and vitality, are also affected by feelings of love. One added benefit is that showing support and affection for loved ones seems to slow the aging process even more than receiving love does."[4]

- Love can also lower your cholesterol levels, improve your immune system, and help protect you against all kinds of disease and premature death.

- Because they can pool their incomes, happily married couples are more financially stable than those who are single. They also tend to have better social support networks. In addition, married people are better equipped as a team to handle life's challenges than are single people, who have to deal with everything on their own. For married people, this can greatly reduce stress.[5]

Like a refreshing oasis in the desert of loneliness, isolation, pain, struggle, and rejection that life can be sometimes, love nourishes health and happiness. It is vital to human well-being to love, and to be loved in return. As George Sand said, "There is only one happiness in life, to love and be loved."

45

Love God
without Being Religious

Let your religion be less of a theory and more of a love affair.

G. K. Chesterton

Building a stronger love relationship with God is similar to strengthening our earthly relationships: it takes time and commitment. But this is where so many of us fail. We make the same mistake that we make with our earthly relationships—we begin with a program! Mom wants to deepen her relationship with her preschooler so she enrolls them both in gymnastics. The husband desires to fall in love with his wife all over again so he sets up a movie date every Friday. Two sisters want to reconnect, so they join a dance class. Although these activities are positive . . . they are just activities. They may bring the people close in proximity and they may be fun, but they will not necessarily be "soul touching."

Soul touching is what happens when two people share their hopes, their disappointments, their joys, and their fears. It requires a willingness to become vulnerable. Each person must risk being known and perhaps ridiculed, or worse, rejected. So many people hide their real selves, and as a result their relationships remain more or less superficial. Is it any wonder that they may try to do the same in their relationship with God and end up with a similar result?

Researchers in the field of neurology have discovered that feelings are generated in certain parts of the right side of the

149

brain and nonemotional actions stem from the brain's left side. Using the technology of the MRI (magnetic resonance imaging) scientists have identified specific regions of the brain that are very active during empathetic and compassionate emotional experiences. For example, when a new mother looks at a picture of her baby, a certain part of her brain becomes highly active, but not when she looks at pictures of other babies. "This care and connection part of the brain shows a profound state of joy and delight that comes from relating to others. This part of the brain does not respond when we perform so-called 'dry' actions, like writing a check, even for a good cause, or performing a service out of duty," explains Dr. Stephen G. Post.[1]

It is so easy to get caught up in *doing* rather than *being*, partially because there are so many good things we can *do* as followers of Jesus. We have wonderful churches with Bible studies of every type. We can join the choir, be on a committee, teach Sunday school, organize programs, do visitation. Doing these things is sometimes motivated by guilt or a sense of obligation aimed at earning or being worthy of God's love. However, if they flow from a heart motivated by love for God, they will be balanced, creative, and powerful, not causing burnout.

But like the husband and wife who are too busy with activities and responsibilities to just *be* with one another, we can become too busy to just *be* with God. There is no longer time to sit and read God's love letters to us or talk to Him without the phone ringing off the hook. We attend all the church services, do our "homework" for the Bible study, get the kids to Sunday school, and make our committee meetings, but we know something is missing. The missing piece is often that our love relationship with God has been squeezed out and our love, peace, joy, and hope have diminished. Our connection has weakened. Many times it is just that we have been too busy with other things, even very good things!

When we are knit closely to God through genuine love for Him, good health and a longer life are often a side benefit. Many studies over the last thirty years have shown the health-enhancing changes that a life of faith can generate. Love for God results in a dynamic prayer life, a desire to worship with others of like faith, and a commitment to care for our bodies fashioned by God Himself. These provide a permeating sense of safety, belonging, and worth. Along with this comes a flood of physiological changes that enhance our health. Yes, there is little doubt that loving God affects our longevity. Here are just a few examples from recent studies:

- Those attending religious services more than once per week have a seven-year survival advantage over those who do not attend.
- Depressed subjects had a 70 percent increase in speed of recovery for each ten-point increase on a religiosity score.
- Those patients with strong beliefs and religious participation showed much better physical functioning and quality of life a year after their surgery.[2]

So how do we renew our love relationship with God? The first and most important step is to acknowledge what has happened. Admit that our relationship with God has cooled, even though to everyone around us we may look busy with the Lord's work and may even be receiving accolades for all the good we do. Talk to God and ask Him for wisdom to know how to simplify your Christian life and strengthen your love relationship with Him. He wants this too and will show you what steps to take.

46

Love Your Liver

A bad liver is to a Frenchman what a nervous breakdown is to an American. Everyone has one and everyone wants to talk about it.

Art Buchwald

Your liver is like a processing plant that performs more than five hundred important functions. It makes proteins and substances that help your blood clot. It makes bile to help you digest your food. It detoxifies harmful substances, including alcohol and certain drugs. Everything that comes into your body through eating, drinking, breathing, and even your skin eventually reaches your liver. It controls metabolism. It stores energy until it is needed. It is your largest organ and the only one that can regenerate itself. But if it is damaged severely enough—scarred through cirrhosis, for example—or becomes infected with a virus such as hepatitis, your days may be numbered. You can live without some of your original parts, but not without your liver.

Liver disease is a significant problem in the United States:

- 30 million Americans, one in every ten, are afflicted with liver-related diseases every year.
- More than 27,000 Americans die each year from chronic liver diseases and cirrhosis.
- There are approximately 4 million people infected with hepatitis C in the United States.
- 8,000 to 10,000 people die of hepatitis C each year.[1]

Symptoms of liver disease differ by person. In some, there may be no symptoms. But the most typical symptoms include: jaundice (yellowing of the skin); darkened urine; nausea; loss of appetite; unusual weight loss or weight gain; vomiting; diarrhea; light-colored stools; abdominal pain in the upper right part of the stomach; malaise, or a vague feeling of illness; generalized itching; varicose veins (enlarged blood vessels); fatigue; hypoglycemia (low blood sugar); low-grade fever; muscle aches and pains; loss of sex drive; depression.[2]

To protect your liver, the Mayo Clinic suggests:

- Drink alcohol in moderation, if at all—two drinks, max, per day for men; women, one.
- Don't mix other drugs with alcohol. Acetaminophen (Tylenol, Excedrin, etc.) can be toxic even if you drink in moderation.
- Avoid contact with other people's blood and body fluids. Hepatitis can be spread via needles, improper cleanup of blood or body fluids, sharing razor blades or toothbrushes, getting tattooed with a dirty needle, or having unsafe sex.
- If you're at increased risk of contracting hepatitis or if you've already been infected with any form of the hepatitis virus, talk to your doctor about getting the hepatitis B vaccine. A vaccine is also available for hepatitis A.
- Only use prescription and nonprescription drugs when you need them, in the recommended doses. Overdoses of over-the-counter medications can be lethal. Talk to your doctor before mixing herbal supplements or prescription or nonprescription drugs.
- Beware of certain supplements that can be toxic to the liver, including kava, comfrey, chaparral, kombucha tea,

pennyroyal, and skullcap. Also avoid high doses of vitamins A, D, E, and K.

- Be careful with aerosol sprays, including aerosol cleaners, insecticides, fungicides, paint, and other toxic chemicals. Wear a mask to keep from inhaling these, and skin covering to keep them from entering through your skin.
- Avoid fatty foods. Your liver makes all the cholesterol your body needs. Eating a well-balanced, nourishing diet rich in whole foods will help your liver do its job properly. Ripe, raw fruits, vegetables, and grains are best; whole food concentrates can fill in the gaps.
- Watch your weight. Even if you don't drink alcohol, obesity can cause a condition called nonalcoholic fatty liver disease, which may include fatty liver, hepatitis, and cirrhosis.[3]

No one is exempt from these rules. A devout young man we will call Bob had a very stressful job. He was quite successful and was rising rapidly in his organization. After each long, hard workday, six days a week, Bob enjoyed having some wine with his wife, who also had a demanding position, while they shared their respective triumphs and not-so-successful moments. While they talked, they often lost track of the time, and Bob often lost track of his wine consumption.

After this pattern had become routine, Bob went in for a physical examination. He was feeling fine and the initial part of his exam was completely normal. But he was unprepared for the results of his blood work. His liver function tests were quite abnormal!

Even after two months of avoiding alcohol, Bob's liver tests were still abnormal, so he agreed to a liver biopsy, which revealed considerable liver damage but thankfully no significant scarring (cirrhosis). Today, a much wiser Bob takes only an occasional drink of wine, and his liver tests have been normal.

47

Mind Your Mouth

The Smiths were shown into the dentist's office, where Mr. Smith made it clear he was in a big hurry.

"No fancy stuff, Doctor," he ordered. "No gas or needles or any of that stuff. Just pull the tooth and get it over with."

"I wish more of my patients were as stoic as you," said the dentist admiringly. "Now, which tooth is it?"

Mr. Smith turned to his wife and said, "Show him, honey."

Only a hundred years ago most people lost their teeth by middle age. Multiple extractions were routine in dentistry. Evidently, folks comforted themselves with the knowledge that they had gained a beautiful smile for life. In addition, they could entertain the children with their "denture tricks," such as making their dentures "talk" as hand puppets or leaving their "teeth" in a jar on the table. Before 1950 it was believed that infection could result from deteriorating teeth. This was the age of replacement, and the advent of anesthesia made a big difference in the pain and suffering associated with extraction of teeth.

However, as dentistry progressed as a specialty, the filling process improved. Most adults were able to keep their teeth for life. Parents taught their children to brush their teeth, and many began going to the dentist regularly. Then in the 1960s came the miracle of fluoride treatments, and fluoride was added to the water supply in many cities, resulting in far fewer cavities.

Eventually, research showed that it was important to keep our teeth at all cost, so crowns were invented and perfected.

At first, dentists were bent on retaining the natural look of the mouth. Bobbie recalls her first crown back in the early '80s and her surprise at seeing her dentist drill a hole to mimic a cavity in her beautiful new crown, then filling it and saying, "You don't want it to look like you have dentures, do you?"

We've come full circle again and all want to have perfect, white teeth. Dental practices offer teeth-whitening and cosmetic dentistry of various kinds. We can buy tooth-whitening toothpaste and in-home teeth-whitening kits at the grocery store. The media has convinced us that we cannot look healthy without white teeth.

But not everyone has blindingly white teeth. At least 36 million people in the United States have periodontal disease. Plaque on teeth can harden into a substance called tartar. Tartar contains bacteria that release acids, causing the delicate tissues around teeth to break down. This causes pockets to form around teeth where bacteria hide and multiply. Signs of periodontal disease, for which one should see a dentist, include bleeding gums during brushing, persistent bad breath, loose or separating teeth, or gums that are red, tender, or swollen.

Tobacco use in any form is a major contributor to gum disease. "Smoking may be responsible for more than half of all cases of periodontal disease among American adults. Other factors that could increase the risk, severity, and speed of development of periodontal disease include medications, stress, genetics, hormonal changes, and poor nutrition."[1]

Recent and ongoing research is demonstrating that nutrition has a lot more to do with dental health than previously thought,[2] and that dental health itself correlates closely with heart disease, diabetes, premature labor, low birth weight babies, peripheral artery disease, stroke, and rheumatoid arthritis.[3]

"Good oral health has recently been linked with longevity. Yet, one of the most common factors associated with infrequent dental checkups is just being male. Men are less likely than women to seek preventive dental care and often neglect their oral health for years. . . . Statistics show that the average man brushes his teeth 1.9 times a day and will lose 5.4 teeth by age 72. If he smokes, he can plan on losing twelve teeth by age 72. Men are also more likely to develop oral and throat cancer and periodontal disease."[4]

Other oral problems also need attention. Grinding teeth while asleep can seriously weaken the teeth. Cold sores and mouth ulcers need attention and usually result from viruses. The biggest danger is that of oral cancer, which is more prevalent in people over 65 years of age. The most common sites for cancer are the tongue, soft palate, floor of the mouth, lips, and gums. If diagnosed early, there is a good chance to be cured, but if it goes undetected it causes pain and disfigurement and eventually death. Each year in the United States 30,000 people are diagnosed with mouth and throat cancer.[5] More than 8,000 people die needlessly each year because they have neglected dental screening and continued with high-risk behaviors such as smoking.[6]

A healthy level of saliva is vital for lubricating our oral cavity, including our teeth, and it washes away acids that attack the teeth. Researchers are using saliva to diagnose diseases such as hepatitis, German measles, pre-term labor, and soon even diabetes. The bottom line is that the mouth is rapidly becoming a window into one's level of health or illness.

Diseases of the mouth are usually associated with poor quality of life. As many as 164 million hours of work are lost yearly due to dental problems.[7] Poor teeth and gums also cause problems with chewing and digesting food, potentially leading to poor nutrition. Conversation can be difficult. It can even hurt to laugh. And then there are the self-esteem issues caused by unsightly teeth, as evidenced when some cover their mouth with each smile. The recent insistence on white, perfect teeth only intensifies our insecurity. But as long as you still have your teeth, be grateful, even if you can't make your dentures "talk" to entertain the kids.

48

Nurture Family Relationships

> The family. We were a strange little band of characters trudging through life sharing diseases and toothpaste, coveting one another's desserts, hiding shampoo, borrowing money, locking each other out of our rooms, inflicting pain and kissing to heal it in the same instant, loving, laughing, defending and trying to figure out the common thread that bound us together.
>
> Erma Bombeck

You may be surprised to know that even your messy, needy, or annoying family members could help you live longer. That is, if you put in the effort to build nurturing relationships so they remain positive influences in your life.

Supportive relationships, especially supportive family relationships, become extremely valuable as we age, while negative family relationships can be detrimental to health. The 2006 book *When I'm 64* explains: "Older parents grow more satisfied with their relationships with their children, who have become adults . . . and the quality of relationships with adult children is strongly associated with parent well-being. . . . Marital satisfaction is also higher in older couples than their younger counterparts . . . and couples (ages 73–93) in a longitudinal study report increasing closeness over time."[1]

Spending time with one's family has become more of a challenge than ever before. The norm is now multigenerational families and even to some degree blended families (where one or both spouses have been married before and bring children to the new relationship). These families do not fit the old-fashioned "Ozzie and Harriet" model. In addition, due to our modern-day mobility, most families actually do not live in the same geographical area, but they can overcome this as needed with the help of modern travel and communications options.

In any case, it is critically important to resolve parent–adult child conflict before grandchildren are born. Research shows that if this conflict exists it may subsequently affect both contact and relationship quality between grandparent and future grandchildren.[2]

Grandparenting has also changed its image and now encompasses people from their 30s up to age 100. More and more seniors are living long and fulfilling lives, seeing their great-great-grandchildren appear on the family scene, bringing the wonderful promise of family triumph and survival. In fact, later life family relationships have emerged as a whole new field of study termed "Family Gerontology."[3] We all have more relatives to deal with for an extended period of time than ever before, so we had better learn the secrets of nurturing family relationships!

The fact that we're a society on the move brings the richness of blending other cultures and races into our family units. A family we know has had the honor and challenge of blending several races and many different geographical backgrounds into their wonderful mix called family. People often ask how they adjusted to the changes. The answer is: *Be willing to change.* Change how you think; change preconceived ideas; change nonbiblical beliefs about right and wrong; change notions about what will make people in your family happy and content; and be willing to change long-held but inaccurate views about what you believe the Bible teaches about a variety of things.

The difference between aging and getting old, wrote Frederic Hudson, is managing life changes so we can be optimally alive, active, and engaged.[4] Change can be refreshing and freeing and makes for happy, vibrant families where all are learners and all have a "kinkeeping" mission.

Families who are determined to stay close and connected make frequent visits a priority and will commit to spending time and money to make them happen. Celebrating family traditions, transitions, and holidays is vitally important. Weddings, birthdays, funerals, and graduations are high on the priority list. Taking fun trips together cements the generations and gives everyone opportunities to change some more!

Siblings become more and more important as we age. Researchers have found that relationships with siblings can contribute to life satisfaction, higher morale, fewer depressive symptoms, psychological well-being, and a greater sense of emotional security in old age.[5] True, if siblings had "rivalries" early in life, these often continue or may resurface later in life. But this can provide the powerful opportunity to journey back to friendship and provide years of fulfillment as well as a valuable role model to the extended family. Experts have ranked sibling relationships as: intimate, congenial, loyal, apathetic, or hostile,[6] and siblings may vacillate between these during different periods in their lives. Sisters usually have the closest bond but also have the most conflict! But sharing a common background and family history can be a powerful magnet and can encourage resolving differences and enjoying the benefits of being truly known and loved. Who else remembers you with braces or was there when . . . !

Strong family relationships are an important foundation for a healthy lifestyle. Nurture them, and never take them for granted.

49

Nurture Something

Gardening and laughing are two of the best things in life you can do to promote good health and a sense of well-being.

David Hobson, *The Mad Gardener*

The word *nurture* means "to nourish, to feed, to help grow." Our words *nurse* and *nursery* have their roots in the word *nurture*. Nursery schools were designed to nurture the young child. Nurseries were designed to nurture plants. And, if you've spent any time in a doctor's office or hospital, you know how nurturing many nurses can be, especially during a time of significant illness or pain.

Anyone who has had the joy of watching vegetables or flowers grow or of caring for a pet understands the emotional satisfaction of nurturing something. Nurturing something is good for your health, as many scientific studies have shown. For example, scientists have known for a long time that gardening has therapeutic and healing qualities, both physically and psychologically. A whole new field of study, horticultural therapy, has developed around the physical and psychological benefits of gardening, and many of those benefits apply also to nurturing our pets.

Gardening and yard work contribute to healthy, active living. Heavy yard work like raking and carrying leaves contributes to both endurance and strengthening muscles, while all those stretches and contortions in the garden can help increase and maintain your flexibility. The most obvious benefit of gardening is exercise, says Dr. Julie Roth of the Wellness Institute at

Northwestern Memorial Hospital in Chicago. "Anyone who has planted trees, created a flower bed from bare lawn, or hauled slate to design a walking path will tell you that dominating Mother Nature is hard work . . . and an enjoyable activity for most people."[1]

Being in a natural environment lowers blood pressure, reduces muscle tension, and increases alpha waves in the brain. In fact, just looking at pictures or videos of nature can reduce stress and lessen negative emotions. No wonder three hundred people who were asked to describe the most healing environment for someone in pain and need of comfort described a place with trees, water, greenery, and stone.[2]

Gardening provides all these health benefits, and in addition the gardeners themselves consume vegetables more frequently than do non-gardeners. Since the consumption of whole foods is one of the most important keys to longevity, enhanced health is one of the gardener's rewards.

The benefits are not just physical; they're also in the mind! Horticultural therapists have discovered that gardening provides a form of emotional expression and release, and it helps people to connect with others. The psychological benefits of being outdoors, working in the sunshine and fresh air, are also clear. One study concluded that those who are involved in gardening find life more satisfying and feel they have more positive things happening in their lives.

People who nurture their pets have similar perspectives and health-enhancing results. "Pets are humanizing," says James Cromwell. "They remind us we have an obligation and responsibility to preserve and nurture and care for all life." Whether it's a dog or cat or goldfish—we're not so sure about rodents, snakes, or frogs, though some seem to prefer them—caring for another being that is more or less entirely dependent on us is healthy.

"Pets have always been a part of my life," Amy said. "I've had several cats and dogs through the years that have brought me deep joy. However, when I moved here, I had to leave my cats, Martha and Mary, behind. I miss the companionship and the joy of caring for something beyond myself. I do, however, have two large flower beds which have become a source of pleasure. One year I grew tomatoes, and last year I planted a rose bush along with my usual annuals. I enjoy getting out on a nice day with my gardening tools, fertilizer, and watering can. What has become an interesting aside, I am actually 'nurturing' the wildlife, as the flowers and vegetables have become food for the rabbits in my yard and the deer that wander through."

Built into most of us is the desire and need to care for something beyond ourselves—whether that be other people, pets, plants, a garden, or the wild animals that come to our backyard feeding stations. The facts are simple:

- Pets provide companionship, help lower blood pressure, reduce stress, prevent heart disease, prevent depression, encourage exercise, help with social support and loneliness, and provide a host of additional benefits.

- Gardening provides exercise; helps lower blood pressure, reduce stress, lessen negative emotions, and increase coping abilities; increases sensory stimulation; provides creative outlets, provides emotional expression and release; and may provide a connection with others if one is involved in a community gardening project. Also, if growing fruits and vegetables is your thing, gardening can reward you with healthy, organically grown produce.

50

Pay the Kindness Forward

No kind action ever stops with itself. One kind action leads to another. Good example is followed. A single act of kindness throws out roots in all directions, and the roots spring up and make new trees. The greatest work that kindness does to others is that it makes them kind themselves.

Amelia Earhart

In the Old Testament, King David took into his palace Mephi-bosheth, the lame son of David's deceased friend, Jonathan (who was the son of Saul, the previous king). It was uncommon to extend such kindness to a possible contender for the throne, but David had loved Jonathan, and to honor that relationship, he chose to extend loving-kindness to Jonathan's son.

In the New Testament, Jesus told the story of "The Good Samaritan" to a group of highly religious folk, including an expert in "the law" (God's law) to clarify what it meant to love your neighbor as yourself. A traveler was robbed and stripped and left for dead. Two supposedly religious, devout Jews—a priest and a Levite—passed by and did nothing. But then a "Samaritan" (despised by and deemed heretics by the Jews to whom the story was told) stopped, bandaged the victim's wounds, took him to an inn, and left the innkeeper with what amounted to a first-century "blank check" to cover the expenses of nursing the traveler back to health. In doing so, the benefactor extended to a total stranger the kindness many would reserve for a blood relative.

Kindness is a spiritual quality that is listed as part of the "fruit of the Spirit" in the New Testament (see Gal. 5:22–23). This suggests that kindness is not necessarily inborn or natural, but a character quality that is often evident in people of faith. For example, if we asked a roomful of people to name the first person who came to mind when we said the word *kindness*, many would name Mother Teresa, who ministered for over forty years to the poor, sick, orphaned, and dying of Calcutta, India. "Kind words can be short and easy to speak," she said, "but their echoes are truly endless." She also said, "Our life of poverty is as necessary as the work itself. Only in heaven will we see how much we owe to the poor for helping us to love God better because of them." In other words, the net result of her kindness was a debt of gratitude to those she helped, for in loving them, she was "loving God better" because, in her own words, "Each one of them is Jesus in disguise."[1]

At this moment, having just been reminded of Mother Teresa's kindness toward the castaways of her world, there is a good chance that you are feeling "the Mother Teresa effect." This phrase was coined by Dr. David McClelland, a prominent researcher of human motivation and health for more than forty years in the late twentieth century. "He and his colleagues had 132 students at Harvard watch a powerful fifty-minute film of Nobel Laureate Mother Teresa aiding the sick and dying of Calcutta. After the film he tested a sample of saliva from each of the students for the level of immunoglobulin A (S-IgA), a vital defense against the cold virus. He found that the students who had seen the film, regardless of whether or not they claimed to admire Mother Teresa's work, showed marked increases in this measure of immune-system function."[2]

In terms of health effects, kindness is a miracle treatment, for it affects the giver, the recipient, and anyone who is a witness.

Serotonin is a chemical in the brain that is related to feeling good. Depression, anxiety, and headaches are often linked to low levels of serotonin. Research shows that being on the receiving end of an act of kindness actually increases your serotonin levels substantially, thus giving you a natural boost of the "feel goods." The great news about giving the gift of kindness to someone is that it's not only the receiver who benefits but also the person who delivers the act of kindness, almost equally. And it doesn't stop there. Anyone who witnesses the act or later hears about it also benefits from elevated levels of serotonin.[3]

Arlene took her friend Ellen to Williamsburg, Virginia, thinking they would do a quick drive-around tour. Arlene had exactly $5 in her purse plus a gasoline card; Ellen had even less. The car died in front of the police station. As Ellen wandered off for a foot tour, Arlene went inside to call an Exxon station. She was happy to discover that the station would repair the vehicle—but not so happy that the work wouldn't be finished until noon the next day! Arlene was sitting on a hard bench outside the courtroom, fighting a panic attack and wondering how she would break the news to Ellen that they may have to beg a jail cell for the night, when a man noticed her, and said, "You look like you've lost your best friend." Fighting back tears, she described her predicament. Without hesitation, the man reached in his pocket, peeled off a number of bills from a roll, and pressed them into her hand with a smile, then walked away. Arlene raced after him. "Wait! I don't know your name or how to pay you back!" He never stopped, but over his shoulder, he said, "I'm Jim, a parole officer here. If you really want to pay it back, you can send it to Jim, care of the Williamsburg Police Department. If not, pay it forward." Arlene nearly danced outdoors to wait to break the news to Ellen that, thanks to a stranger's kindness, they had enough for a room and food until the car was fixed. Arlene still recalls this event thankfully, and tries to "pay the kindness forward" whenever she can.

51

Play More

Men do not quit playing because they grow old; they grow old because they quit playing.[1]

Oliver Wendell Holmes

Want to improve your quality of life? Play more. Stuart Brown of the Institute of Play compares those who play and those who don't: "What do Nobel Laureates, innovative entrepreneurs, artists and performers, well-adjusted children, happy couples and families, and the most successfully adapted mammals have in common? They play enthusiastically throughout their lives. What common denominator is shared by mass murderers, abused children, burnt-out employees, depressed mothers, caged animals, and chronically worried students? Play is rarely or never a part of their lives."[1]

If "all work and no play makes Jack a dull boy," where does that leave most of us? If your life is dull and you want it full, perhaps you would do well to work harder at playing and not so hard at working. Americans seem to consider "productivity" as close to the highest good. We work like slaves for a little paid time off, while in much of Europe, ample time off has long been a given. Though things are changing there, it remains true that while Americans live to work, Europeans work to live . . . and to play.

"Play is extremely important for humans from birth to death," says Marianne St. Clair. "Play is not meant to be just for children. It is a form of release and connection that can tap the creativity and can allow you the chance to connect with the child inside you. Play is a state of mind, but it is also a state of body, emotion, and spirit. Yes . . . it is something you do (playing games, swinging, exercising), but it is also something you watch others do, and gain pleasure from simply watching. It is often described as a time when we feel most alive, yet it is something we take for granted and may forget to do. It can be entirely positive, or can be dramatic. Play can be used in many ways to not only stimulate creativity, but as a way to transform negative emotions. We are hardwired as adults to engage in play, and it is crucial to our vitality to spend time with play each day."[2]

Feelings associated with play include delight, clarity, confidence, serenity, and timelessness, according to psychiatrist Mihaly Csikszentmihalyi. This set of feelings suggests total engagement of the person involved—fully alive and immersed in the present. What better way to renovate, rejuvenate, and forget the stress for a while? There are lifelong benefits also, starting on the playground, including the development of social skills, communication, and cooperation. Team games include responsibility, teamwork, determination, and shared happiness when the team wins.[3]

Even playing board games or cards or doing crossword puzzles has health benefits. A study published in the *New England Journal of Medicine* found that challenging your brain with mentally stimulating activities helps stave off dementia.[4]

Play is as necessary to our health and well-being as is eating right and getting enough sleep. We play to relax, get away from the daily grind, learn, create, feel challenged, pass time, have fun, be with others, compete or watch others compete, and a host of other reasons. Play is important outside of work and at work as well. Quality work is dependent on the well-being of workers, not on the amount of time spent working. Wise employers have learned to incorporate leisure activities into the work environment by providing exercise equipment, weight-loss groups, massage therapy, basketball courts, chess tournaments, walking groups, and other activities. They have found that a few minutes of "play" each day can increase energy and thus productivity. A little play increases well-being among employees, triggers creativity and clearer thinking, and renews hope. It just plain makes work more enjoyable and fun!

On a personal level, don't work too hard at trying to play, or the result will be less healthful, for sure. For example, instead of walking for exercise, make it fun. Play with the dog as you go. Count how many cars pass by, how many people you see wearing red hats, how many yards have flowers, how many different sounds you hear. Blow bubbles into the breeze . . . anything to get your mind off issues that may be weighing you down. Or, if your family loves to camp, sometime in the winter, set up your tents and sleeping bags indoors. Turn off the electric lights and use candles or an electric lantern, cook hot dogs in your fireplace, make S'mores and hot chocolate, sing camping songs or tell some tall tales or jokes, and then on the wings of faith and trust and pixie dust, drift off to dreamland.

Make play a priority as you grow older. In addition to adding to a good healthy lifestyle and increased longevity, you'll be emulating some pretty good role models. Michel de Montaigne wrote, "There is nothing more notable in Socrates than that he found time, when he was an old man, to learn music and dancing, and thought it time well spent."[5]

52

Practice Generosity

Giving is the secret of a healthy life. Not necessarily money, but whatever a person has of encouragement, sympathy and understanding.

John D. Rockefeller

Giving money is only part of the health-enhancing quality we call generosity. In other words, you don't have to be rich to be generous, though if you are generous with whatever you have, including your time, talents, work, or knowledge, you will become "rich" in relationships and love. As Jesus taught, "Give, and it will be given to you. A good measure, pressed down, shaken together and running over, will be poured into your lap. For with the measure you use, it will be measured to you" (Luke 6:38).

True generosity involves giving from the heart to try to help someone else. According to Allan Luks, helpers are healthier overall. "What appears to be at work here is a combination of factors, varying in weight and frequency of occurrence, which include:

- the possibility of strengthening immune-system activity
- decrease of both the intensity and the awareness of physical pain
- activation of the emotions that are vital to the maintenance of good health
- reduction of the incidence of attitudes, such as chronic hostility, that negatively arouse and damage the body

- the multiple benefits to the body's systems provided by stress relief."[1]

A generous act is accompanied by "feel good" hormones. You might even call it a brain cell "oxytocin" bath. Paul J. Zak of Claremont Graduate University gave doses of oxytocin or a placebo to participants who were asked to make a one-time decision to split money they were given with a stranger. "Those who were given oxytocin offered 80 percent more money than those given the placebo. Oxytocin specifically and powerfully affected generosity using real money when participants had to think about another's feelings. Zak's research explains why in 2005 over 65 million Americans volunteered to help charities. Ninety-six percent of the volunteers said that one of their motivations was feeling compassionate toward other people."[2]

Why people give is really known only to God, who, by the way, "loves a cheerful giver." We say this because we can even fool ourselves about our motives for giving. For example, when we gave a dollar to that street person standing on the corner holding the "homeless" sign, was it an act of compassion or pity, or was it to protect ourselves from emotional discomfort later had we just driven on by? Sometimes our giving can be driven by guilt, as when the preacher says that really spiritual people "tithe." By contrast, in one church that we (Bobbie and Jim) attended, the pastor would actually ask that those in attendance *not* contribute at offering time unless they could do so out of a heart of joy, caring, and thanksgiving. That church's needs were always met.

A recent study involving 125 participants discovered that "thoughts related to God cultivate cooperative behavior and generosity."[3] The task was for one group to unscramble sentences with spiritual words versus a control group whose scrambled sentences had no spiritual words. The participants then played a game that involved sharing with an anonymous recipient. Those primed with the religious terms were much more generous—68 percent of subjects from the religiously primed group allocated their money portion to anonymous strangers, compared to 22 percent in the other group.

As far as we can see, there are two kinds of people in the world—givers and takers. Givers will stop and share a few moments, even if they really should be going. Takers never stop, unless they want to ask for something. Givers help others learn a new sport or game or hobby or vocation. For takers, there's no future in such unproductive activities. Givers volunteer to help organizations, without stipulations like "I don't do windows." Takers infiltrate charitable organizations, take control, and then ask givers to do the toilets in addition to the windows.

Givers are satisfied to give, asking nothing in return. They are generally healthier and happier than takers, who are always anxiously looking over their shoulders to see who might be coming along to take away what they themselves have taken from others.

"You wish to be happy? Loved? Safe? Secure? You want to turn to others in tough times and count on them? You want the warmth of true connection? You'd like to walk into the world each day knowing that this is a place of benevolence and hope? Then I have one answer: give. Give daily, in small ways, and you will be happier. Give and you will be healthier. Give and you will live longer."[4]

53

Practice Safe Sex

Bob and Fred, both widowers in their 80s, are discussing Bob's plan to remarry. The fiancée is 42. Fred says, "You know, Bob, making love at your age with someone her age could be dangerous, don't you think?" Bob winks and replies, "If she dies, she dies."

Author unknown

Our sexuality is one of God's gifts, meant to be valued and enjoyed within the marriage relationship. The power of the sexual experience to build a strong emotional bond enhancing all other aspects of a couple's relationship has been proven again and again. Recently, scientists have also learned that a healthy sex life can not only enhance our quality of life but also affect longevity. The British National Health Service claims that "'sexercise' will not only lower the risk of heart attack but will help people live longer . . . the endorphins released will stimulate immune system cells, which also target illness like cancer, as well as wrinkles. . . . About 300 calories an hour can be burned as well as getting a healthy workout for the heart and lungs. Healthy bones and muscles, and a feeling of well-being are, they say, a guaranteed result of the production of extra estrogen and testosterone hormones which sex engenders."[1]

Information gathered from 3,005 Americans ages 57 to 85 showed without a doubt that they possess vitality and interest in sexuality well into their later years. The study also showed that seniors regard intimacy as an important part of life, despite a high rate of bothersome sexual problems.[2]

God's purpose for marriage is for sexuality to enhance general well-being as well as the marriage relationship. A recent AARP survey of 1,700 baby boomers confirmed that most "remained steadfastly traditional when it came to fidelity. . . . The survey also found many saying that good spirits, good health, close ties with friends, and family and spiritual well-being were more important than sex. Sixty-three percent of men and women with partners described themselves as either extremely or somewhat satisfied with their sex lives."[3]

When sexually transmitted disease (STD) enters the picture, sex can turn from life enhancing to deadly. STDs are infections that are transmitted during any type of sexual encounter; some are spread by kissing. Although treatment is available for many STDs, others are not yet curable. You may believe that STDs are a problem for the young. However, according to the Centers for Disease Control (CDC), people 45, 50, and older are "experiencing staggering increases in STD transmission, particularly in women. . . . People in their 40s contract STDs at twice the rate of people in their 20s."[4]

The list of diseases that can be transmitted sexually include: bacterial vaginosis, chlamydia, genital HPV infection, genital herpes, gonorrhea, hepatitis B, lymphogranuloma venereum, pelvic inflammatory disease, HIV, syphilis, and trichomoniasis.

Phil and Linda went through a rocky period in their marriage as the kids left home one by one and Linda was having health problems. Struggling to find distraction and comfort, Phil succumbed to the advances of his personal trainer and had a brief affair with her before he reconciled with his wife. Guilt ridden and concerned about possible disease, he went to his physician for a checkup that confirmed he had contracted human papillomavirus (HPV). Further tests confirmed he had already spread it to his wife.

HPV causes genital warts in men and women. Each year, 6.2 million new cases are diagnosed. The CDC warns that by age 50 at least 80 percent of women will have contracted HPV.[5] There is no known cure, but treatment is available. However, if left untreated, HPV can cause precancerous changes in men and women and even become a full-blown cancer.

As older Americans live longer and healthier and men enjoy increased virility with drugs such as Viagra, the CDC is concerned that the number of STDs is rising in the elderly. "During the last decade," they report, "HIV cases have risen 500 percent among senior citizens and AIDS cases among people over 50 have risen from 1,600 in 1975 to 9,000 in 2003. Now nearly 27 percent of people living with AIDS in America are 50 and older."[6]

Why such a huge increase? The answer includes these factors:

1. A longer, healthier lifespan allows for sexual behavior later in life.
2. Senior citizens may not be as cautious as younger people, who have been well educated regarding sex.
3. Many seniors do not consider the necessity of protection, since pregnancy is not an issue.
4. With the advent of Viagra and similar medications, more men are resuming an active (sometimes overactive) sex life.
5. Dating has become more socially acceptable following the death of a spouse or divorce.
6. Dating multiple partners has become more popular in America.

7. Patients may feel uncomfortable discussing sexuality with doctors; likewise, some doctors may feel the same in relation to older patients.

Jane contracted HIV in the mid-1980s; then founded the National Association on HIV over 50 (www.hivoverfifty.org). She encourages teens to explain safe sex to their elders. Several universities have even included this assignment in their classes on gerontology. So if your grandchild or the teen down the street attempts to pass on their knowledge about safe sex, be thankful that they care and have learned that parents are vulnerable too. Meanwhile, celebrate your sexuality and its benefits for a longer, fulfilled life, confining it to the best and safest context—marriage to an uninfected spouse.

54

Pray 24/7

Pray without ceasing.

1 Thessalonians 5:17 KJV

Suppose you could have the full attention of your closest friend anytime, day or night. Not only could you share what is on your heart with them but they would respond by partnering with you in whatever concerns you—helping, supporting, advising, encouraging. Although no human can begin to accomplish this level of personal involvement with you and your needs, God can and He does.

God is able and willing to change our situations as needed, to heal and give hope where there is none, and to enter into our pain and grief to provide comfort. Christians (literally, "Christ's ones") are never alone because Christ's Father, God, stands with us in adversity, sharing our burdens and sorrows and also our joys. Knowing we are not alone as we live day to day provides a sense of serenity and security that is surely a context for optimal health.

According to Dr. Marty Sullivan, "People who pray or meditate experience the *relaxation response*: a drop in blood pressure, heart rate, and levels of stress hormones, such as cortisol."[1]

A Duke University Medical Center study concluded that even occasional private prayer and Bible study helped people live healthier and longer lives. Researcher Harold Koenig, MD, reports that "this is one of the first studies showing that people who pray live longer."[2] In another context Dr. Koenig writes, "The person who prays is less stressed. He becomes less anxious, and his blood pressure and pulse improve."

What we mean by "prayer" is simply communicating with our heavenly Father. The Scriptures mention this more than two hundred times. One of the amazing privileges of being a child of God is that we are connected with a God who is never too busy to listen and who wants us to "pray continually" (1 Thess. 5:17). If praying were just saying words or repeating phrases that somebody else put into a "prayer book," fulfilling this instruction would not be possible. It is only possible to pray continually if prayer is an attitude of the heart—an attitude of worship, praise, thanksgiving, submission, and humility that wants what God wants and longs that His will would be done on earth as it is in heaven. In the words of John Bunyan, "When you pray, rather let your heart be without words, than your words without heart."

One of our physician friends wrote:

I have had some of my best times beside a meadow stream, enjoying the pattern of the ripples of the clear water along the pebbles and watching ducks float by. I especially like birds and the wonder of their freedom in flight. My thoughts of the Creator soar as I watch the birds do aerial stunts. I enjoy praying at such times when walking through the forest.

Recently I rode my bicycle to Willamette Mission Park. Blue flowers lined the paths, and in places yellow buttercups with bright golden trimming gathered and were gently being blown in the wind to and fro as if to illuminate different petal castings upon the black-eyed Susans in the background. Out in Hagg Lake the powder puffed cottonwood seeds summersault along the surface of the water to the whim of the gentle breeze. There were kayakers making group efforts to learn how to swamp their boats and escape underwater, and on shore, a group of children splashing on the bank, and a flock of Canada geese low flying closer together than the Blue Angels squadron. It seemed I could have reached up and touched their feathers if they had flown a bit closer my way. At the end of my time praying in God's handiwork I am always able to say with more surety, "Yes, it is well with my soul."[3]

Sometimes we send up sentence prayers. Sometimes we pray as we walk or work. Sometimes we spend a few minutes alone with God at the start and end of our day. Sometimes we thank Him before meals or sing a prayer to Him as we make our way somewhere. Sometimes we ask forgiveness when we have strayed from His way. Sometimes we join with other believers to pray for help or healing or other concerns. The method does not matter as much as having our heart and mind focused on Him. This is what He desires and what prayer is all about—a spiritual connection that is open 24/7.

One of our friends shared, "I have an author friend, who is also a local pastor's wife. I read a book of hers years ago and thought: *If I have a question about this book, I can just call my friend, the author.* I remember thinking about what a gift that was and how blessed I was, since most readers are unable to simply make a phone call to an author. Later the Lord said to me, 'When you are reading My book and have a question, you don't even have to pick up the telephone! You can simply pray and I'll explain it to you.' It was one of those aha moments in my life!"

We trust that if you've never experienced such an aha moment, you will do so soon, and that over time you'll learn how to keep that particular line of communication open 24/7.

55

Prevent Accidents

Accidental death in America is a silent epidemic; with one person dying from an accident every five minutes. Unintentional injury is one of the most serious public health issues facing the country.

Alan McMillan, National Safety Council
President and CEO

There is a good reason we often say to each other in parting, "See you soon and take care." In September 2007, new data showed that accidental deaths in the U.S. are increasing at a rate of more than 20 percent over a ten-year period! Yet the leading causes of accidental injury and death in this country are all preventable.[1]

Killer #1: Motor vehicle accidents continue to be the number one accidental killer. Stiffer penalties, better education, more stop signs and traffic lights, and law enforcement have improved in most states, but U.S. drivers continue to be dangerous and distracted. Speeding and failure to wear seat belts are often blamed for deaths. Road rage is often cited as a cause for high risk behaviors. Increasing numbers of sleep-deprived drivers are driving drowsy. Cell phone use while driving is another culprit. In states where cell phone use while driving is still permitted, you will see drivers laughing, shouting, and waving their phones in the air as they converse while driving along. "Texting" while driving has dwarfed concerns over distractingly loud stereos.

Killer #2: The second overall cause of accidental death is poisoning from overdoses of prescription and illegal drugs. This is the fastest rising cause of accidental death, with a 5 percent increase in 2005 alone! "While the largest numerical increase in overdoses is among white men—up nearly 6,000 in 10 years—poisoning death rates are increasing the most among white women—up more than 300 percent over 10 years."[2]

One reason for the increase is the large number of the elderly taking medications. Although pharmacists and physicians diligently try to educate older patients about dosing and side effects, failing eyesight, impaired memory, and poor hearing can sometimes cause them to make tragic mistakes. There are some simple remedies, including the use of plastic boxes designed to contain each day's set of pills, which visiting nurses, friends, and family can monitor without being intrusive.

But even young people who take multiple prescriptions are at risk for drug interactions or a deadly overdose. In January 2008, we all were shocked when the death of 28-year-old movie star Heath Ledger was ruled an accidental overdose of prescription drugs. The official report stated that Ledger died from acute intoxication from the combined effects of six prescription drugs.[3] His heartbroken family issued this sobering statement: "Heath's accidental death serves as a caution to the hidden dangers of combining prescription medication, even at low dosage."

Killer #3: In 2004 alone, 18,807 deaths from falls in the United States were recorded by the National Safety Council. The majority occurred as people were just walking around in their homes. Since 1992, the death rate from injuries occurring in the home or community has increased by 30 percent.[4] Falls occur in many ways—tripping over the dog or rug; falling off the bed or chair; slipping in the shower or on ice in the driveway; tumbling down the stairs; or plunging off a roof.

Killer #4: The fourth major cause of accidental death is choking. As we age, choking becomes more of a risk due to factors such as a narrowing of the esophagus. That combined with poorly aligned teeth or dentures may cause seniors to chew food improperly; this can result in food becoming lodged in the throat. Fortunately, the majority of the time, a bystander taking quick action with the Heimlich maneuver can free the blockage. Holiday dinners and eating a hot dog at the ballpark are examples of times we should be especially careful to chew our food well.

Killer #5: Drowning is the number five cause nationally of accidental death. In 1995, over 3,500 people died by drowning in the United States; about 1,500 were children. Most infants drowned in bathtubs, toddlers in swimming pools, and older children in various freshwater locations like rivers and lakes. Alcohol use is involved in up to half of adolescent and adult drowning deaths.[5] When warnings are obeyed and safety tips followed, most drownings are preventable.

These five causes account for 83 percent of all accidental deaths in the United States. In addition to the 113,000 accidental deaths reported in 2005, 24 million nonfatal accidents occurred during the same year.[6] A nonprofit group based in a Chicago suburb recently estimated the annual cost of accidents in the

United States to be $625.5 billion (including wage and productivity losses, medical expenses, and motor vehicle damage).[7]

It may seem that the world is filled with warnings: cross the street only at the walkway; slow down, sharp curve ahead; do not pass; beware of falling rocks; high surf; do not leave a burning candle unattended; and so forth.

Some people have thought that such warnings may apply to everyone else but not to them, and they're dead as a result. We think that it's far better to view these warnings as voices of your larger family, humanity, who are trying to keep you safe and sound instead of having to list your cause of death as "accidental."

56

Remember Who's in Charge of Your Health

"Doc, my sugar is 180 to 200 every time I test it."

"Have you made those diet changes we discussed?"

"I tried, but I can't seem to give up my Cokes and donuts. And eat raw vegetables? My fishing buddies just laughed and said they wouldn't want to be me."

"Well, you need to understand that your food choices are shortening your life!"

"Come on, Doc. You gotta have some other ideas . . . just give me some pills or something to fix it."

> Dr. Jim has had numerous conversations
> like this with patients.

When Jim and Bobbie were just graduating from their training programs in the early '60s, health care was totally different. The popular TV show *Marcus Welby, M.D.*, depicted it well. The kind, all-knowing, grandfatherly family doctor cared for you and managed all your health problems. He always knew what should be done and patients looked to him for his sage advice, which they followed without question. This was the golden age of medical "paternalism," meaning that the "pater" (father) directed your steps and made all your most important decisions for you.

In the past, most families had their own generalist or family doctor who often was a valued friend caring for the entire family. From grandfather to newborn, all were entrusted into his competent hands. In cases where families came upon hard times and could not pay, he gladly accepted a nice chicken, some fresh corn or tomatoes from the garden, or some free plumbing as payment. House calls were commonplace and your friendly, though care-worn doctor would show up at your door in the middle of the night if you called. He performed surgery, delivered babies, and even counseled your troubled teen.

Today, Dr. Welby is no more. For the most part, doctors are "providers" of health care and patients are "consumers." Many are very educated consumers, in terms of health issues, since so much information is readily available on the Internet. Some have health insurance, but many do not. Either way, expenditures on health care have surpassed the value of your grandma's whole garden or whole chicken coop by a significant margin.

Most patients who are old enough to have access to Medicare find that the cost of health care is still more than they had planned for. In a recent survey by the Kaiser Family Foundation, Americans fret more about their health care costs than they do about losing a job, paying the mortgage, or becoming a victim of terrorism.[1] In other words, becoming a victim of disease poses a greater perceived threat to most people than just about anything. Surely, something must change!

Mary Jo Kreitzer has an answer: "YOU are the one who can make the biggest impact on your own health . . . and here is the reason why," she writes. "The health care system (drugs, care providers, and hospitals) affects only about 10 percent of our health. The remaining 90 percent of health outcomes is determined by factors over which health care providers have little or no control, such as lifestyle choices, social conditions, and the physical environment."[2]

To maintain and improve our health, we need to not only make good lifestyle choices but also get the best health care we can. Even those of us without health insurance can assemble a health care team with ourselves as the captain. "Nurse practitioners can frequently offer the same care as a doctor, at a lower rate," says Allison Beard, spokesperson for the American College of Nurse Practitioners. "Nurse practitioners fill a needed void in the health care system today. Research comparing nurse practitioners with physicians shows that nurses tend to spend more time with patients, charge less, and do just as good a job of diagnosing problems."[3]

You might also consider adding a parish/congregational nurse to your health care team. Many churches across the United States have parish nurses on their staff who run screening clinics and offer education classes. Parish nurses also help their parishioners navigate the health care system and act as an advocate when someone is hospitalized. Bobbie has been a parish nurse at different times in her career and believes parish nurse services can be beneficial in many circumstances.

While nothing can replace mainline medical care for things such as infection, fractures, bleeding, or issues requiring surgery, for many chronic conditions or stress-related diseases, you may want to consider acupuncture or massage therapy. Acupuncture can be effective for chronic pain as well as postoperative nausea and vomiting, among other things. Sometimes massage therapy can loosen up muscle spasms that nothing else can help.

Taking charge of your health does not mean turning your back on all options offered by medical professionals. Rather, your goal is to assemble a team of qualified allies with special talents ready to assist you in maintaining your health. You may even find that this approach works better for you, personally, than when the whole town was sharing one "Dr. Welby."

57

Save Your Skin

A patient recently told me that, though I am 52, I had the skin of a 40-year-old. When I told my wife, Deb, she said, "Give it back; you're getting it all wrinkled."

Robert W. Martin III, MD, MAR (author of this chapter)

Unlike any other organ or system within the body, the skin's aging process is readily visible. The skin ages internally and externally. The skin of a person never exposed to the sun would develop a smooth, unblemished surface. External factors (smoking, pollution, and especially sunlight) cause 90 percent of the wrinkles, 100 percent of the discoloration, and most skin cancers.

As much as 50 percent of a person's total sun exposure occurs before the age of 25. Without protection from the sun's rays, just a few minutes of exposure each day over the years can cause noticeable changes to the skin. Damage is generally most pronounced in fair-skinned individuals, especially in those who have had ample occupational or recreational exposure to sunlight throughout their lives. There is no safe tan! Repeated use of tanning beds doubles the risk of skin cancer, especially melanoma.

One blistering childhood sunburn doubles the lifetime risk for skin cancer. Children under six months of age should be protected by clothing and shade. Between six months and two years, a broad-spectrum sunblock, such as titanium dioxide or zinc oxide should be used. After the age of two, chemical sunscreens may be applied.

Sunscreens should be broad-spectrum (protecting against UVA and UVB rays) with an SPF 15 or higher—this applies to all ages. Sunscreens should be amply applied at least twenty minutes before sun exposure and reapplied every two hours—year-round. Contrary to popular belief, sunscreen does not cause vitamin D deficiency, since it only takes two to five minutes of sun exposure for maximum natural production of vitamin D. Avoiding sun exposure between 10:00 a.m. and 4:00 p.m., wearing long pants and long-sleeved shirts of tightly woven synthetic fabrics, gloves, and a broad-brimmed hat are also recommended.

The most common malignancy in women ages 25–34 is melanoma. Men over the age of 50 are at the highest risk for melanoma, but it can affect anyone, of any age. Melanoma is more common in people who had severe childhood sunburns and who have fair skin, more than one hundred moles, a family history of melanoma, weakened immune system, or unusual moles called dysplastic nevi. The most frequent sites for melanoma are the upper back, chest, abdomen, and lower legs. Caught early, melanoma is curable. Ignored, it can be fatal. I teach patients this melanoma warning signs acrostic:

Asymmetry of a mole—i.e., the halves do not match.

Borders are irregular, notched, or scalloped.

Color variation is present with different shades of brown, tan, or black.

Diameter is larger than a pencil eraser.

Evolving changes in size, shape, color, elevation, bleeding, itching, or crusting of moles.

During our 40s and 50s our skin begins to thin and become less elastic. There are more brown spots and wrinkles. The most likely cause is sun damage. Over-the-counter "wrinkle" creams and lotions do little or nothing to reverse wrinkles. At this time, only prescription tretinoin cream and certain lasers have been approved by the FDA to treat sun-damaged or aging skin. Dermatologists can treat wrinkling with injectable fillers/botulinum toxin, dermabrasion, laser resurfacing, chemical peeling, microdermabrasion, and topical treatments.

During our 60s and 70s the tip of the nose droops, wrinkles deepen, our ears elongate, our eyelids fall, jowls form, and the upper lip disappears while the lower lip protrudes. No, you're not becoming a werewolf; it's just gravity. Once-flat brown spots now become raised and scaly, blood vessels dilate, and permanent brown spots occur not only on the face but on the neck, chest, arms, and legs—permitting grandchildren hours of "connect-the-dot" entertainment, hopefully with a washable magic marker!

Two of the most common problems during this stage are the risk of non-melanoma skin cancers and dry skin. Dry skin affecting the back, lower legs, and arms results from loss of sweat and oil glands and thinning of the skin. Low humidity, dehydration, sun exposure, smoking, stress, diabetes, kidney disease, certain medications, and overuse of soaps, antiperspirants, perfumes, or hot baths will make the problem worse. My "Rule of 3s" is:

1. Tub bath/shower no more than 3/week;
2. Water 3–5 degrees above body temperature (i.e., tepid water);
3. Bathe for less than 3–5 minutes;
4. Pat dry, leaving "beads of water," and apply emollient within 3 minutes;
5. Apply body lotion 3 additional times per day.

Non-melanoma skin cancer affects one in five Americans and occurs most commonly on sun-exposed areas. Skin cancer risk is greatest for fair-skinned "frecklers" with a past history of significant sun exposure. Basal cell carcinomas are usually small, fleshy bumps or nodules on the head and neck. Squamous cell carcinomas are tumors that may appear as nodules or as red, scaly patches that can develop into large masses and spread to other parts of the body. Any persistent open sore or red patch; new, shiny, pink, or crusty bump; or a scarlike area (occurring where there has been no surgery or trauma) is cause for alarm and requires evaluation by a dermatologist.

While aging is not for sissies, Shakespeare wrote, "With mirth and laughter let old wrinkles come."

58

Seek Solitude

Our language has wisely sensed the two sides of man's being alone. It has created the word "loneliness" to express the pain of being alone. And it has created the word "solitude" to express the glory of being alone.

Paul Johannes Tillich

Even the youngest child understands the pain of loneliness. But as an adult, you can experience loneliness if your last child just left for college, you've lost someone you love by divorce or death, or you're just spending a particularly endless Saturday afternoon by yourself when everyone else seems to be more happily engaged. You may suddenly notice that your arthritis is flaring up, or your few gray hairs have mobilized into a solid coalition, and you obviously need a little *nap* instead of your customary walk around the block.

While many studies have linked loneliness and ill health, recent research conducted at UCLA by Steve Cole, PhD, and associates found genetic evidence for this effect. "Compared with their socially connected peers, the lonely had overactive genes that promote inflammation and cell growth," wrote Miranda Hitti in her analysis of this study. "Lonely people also had underactive genes that control inflammation and cells' life cycle. Those genetic patterns may show why chronic loneliness has long been linked to poorer health and accelerated aging."[1]

Loneliness and solitude create different emotions depending on how you view and value being alone, and how you choose to use that time. Choosing to spend time with yourself and God opens the door to recommitment to old goals, dreams for tomorrow, inner healing, or creativity.

Philosopher and writer Henry David Thoreau hunkered down by the shores of Walden Pond. Aviator Anne Morrow Lindberg found her muse at the edge of the ocean. She wrote, "The loneliness you get by the sea is personal and alive. It doesn't subdue you and make you feel abject. It's stimulating loneliness." Both sought out and were solaced by solitude.

189

In their abstract of "Solitude: An Exploration of Benefits of Being Alone," the article's authors say:

Historically, philosophers, artists, and spiritual leaders have extolled the benefits of solitude; currently, advice on how to achieve solitude is the subject of many popular books and articles. Seldom, however, has solitude been studied by psychologists, who have focused instead on the negative experiences associated with being alone, particularly loneliness. Solitude, in contrast to loneliness, is often a positive state—one that may be sought rather than avoided. In this article, we examine some of the benefits that have been attributed to solitude—namely, freedom, creativity, intimacy, and spirituality.[2]

Solitude cannot be bought—for example, by building a "studio" down by the creek on the back forty. Nor can it be manufactured, though some organizations promote their programs as events through which participants can find solitude. One such program cost $250 and required sharing a room with a total stranger so the 450 participants *couldn't* speak to each other but instead could spend quality time alone. The program was sold out.

François Fénelon (1651–1715) was a French mystic who was exiled after rising to one of the highest offices in the French court. He wrote, "Sometimes the annoyances that make you long for solitude are better for producing humility than the most complete solitude could be. Do not seek God as if He were far off in an ivory castle. He is found in the middle of the events of your everyday life. Listen to the voice of God in silence. Be willing to accept what He wants to show you. God will show you everything you need to know. Be faithful to come before Him in silence. When you hear the still, small voice within, it is time to be silent."[3]

59

Simplify Your Life

If over-involvement, clutter, and busyness are the rulers of our lives, then it's snuffing out our happiness, our purpose and our joy.

H. Norman Wright

For most of us, life is plagued by "too manys"—too many commitments, too many tasks, too many bills, too many boxes in the garage, too many shoes! Many of these things are good, even admirable in themselves. And even though there is little direct scientific evidence to date examining the health effect of simplifying, constantly having too many commitments, tasks, bills, boxes, or shoes can deplete our energy and time and leave us exhausted from working so hard to pay the bills, confused about what we really want, and chronically distressed and/or depressed, all of which can be detrimental to health and longevity—as explained elsewhere in this book. This problem is so prevalent that if you Google "simplify your life," you'll find over 220,000 entries online.

The place to start is not by cluttering your mind with advice from thousands of sources but to begin at the beginning, specifically with your value system, for this controls most of your decisions. One by one, your decisions control your direction in life, and ultimately, whether you end up "traveling light" or trying to tote enough baggage to bring a horse to its knees. Or, are you trying to tote the horse too?

191

Dave's good friend Dr. Richard Swenson has written extensively on this subject, including his books *Margin* and *The Overload Syndrome*. In the latter he describes how he and his wife decided to simplify their life:

> I will never forget the evening when Linda and I, on our living room floor, decided it was time to make substantive changes. Together we took out a pad of paper and sat down before the fireplace. "Let's start by pretending everything in our lives is written on this paper," I suggested. "Every attitude, every activity, every belief, every influence. Then let's erase it all. Tear up the paper and throw it in the fire. Wipe the slate clean. . . ."
>
> It was an exciting evening. An exhilarating sense of freedom swept over us. As we wrestled control of our lives away from the world, we felt the elephant slipping off our backs. . . . Our redesigned life was simpler. That decision reduced our income significantly, but the freedom, the time, the rest, and the balance have been well worth it. We have never looked back.[1]

Every person has a unique core system of values. The main issue here, though, is that if your decisions are not in tune with your value system, there will be tension and stress in your life, even if it's only some indefinable background noise.

Once you have identified your core values, you can begin to simplify. Everything you do and all the possessions you have accumulated (or plan to buy) can be viewed through the lens of your values. At first, deciding which clothing or recreation equipment to keep may feel like you are deciding which family member to give away—for example, your 30-year-old son's first teddy bear or the blouse your grandmother bought you forty years ago.

The number of activities you're involved with may also seem, at first, hard to limit. For many people, the more socially involved they are, the more invitations they have to get involved with new things, most of which are good in themselves. But too many good things can produce overload too. Follow Dr. Swenson's example, and start with a blank sheet and ask yourself: *If we weren't involved with anything at all, which activities would we choose?*

Jim and Bobbie embarked on a life of simplification a number of years ago. After practicing medicine for years and having raised their family, they were beginning the fourth lap of life, that of phasing down. This journey soon took them surprisingly to an exciting life on the road as they did temporary medical work around the country, going where there was a need for several months at a time. They loved the life and the opportunity to help in times of need and began shedding "baggage" as they went. "It was hard to part with the things we loved," admits Bobbie, "but there was also a sense of freedom in traveling light. We were amazed at how little we really needed." Six years later, Bobbie and Jim continued to live on the road. Their usual "home" was a one-bedroom, furnished apartment, with one closet for clothes. The time they have regained has enabled them to live life in the slower lane and do more of the things they love.

It is also possible to simplify your spiritual life. Laura wrote:

One snowy Sunday morning as we were trying to get our three small children ready for church, I felt a pounding headache creeping toward my temple. Rushing to find the hats, which should have been in the basket by the door, I stumbled and fell headlong into the railing. Tears welled up in my eyes and, as the children stood wide-eyed around me, I felt totally overwhelmed. When my husband came in from dutifully shoveling the snowdrift away from the car, we just looked at each other, clouded in discouragement. This was the beginning of a wholehearted effort to simplify and bring balance and sanity back into our lives. The chaos of our life had crept into our spiritual life as well. Somehow, even going to the church we loved and attending a weekly Bible study had become just one more thing on our to-do list.

193

If this sounds familiar, isn't it time to simplify? As Dr. Swenson says, "A life voluntarily chosen and lived in freedom; a life uncluttered and natural; a life that is focused, diligent, and disciplined; a life characterized by creativity and spiritual authenticity—is not this a healthy life?"[2]

60

Stay Active

We are under exercised as a nation. We look instead of play. We ride instead of walk. Our existence deprives us of the minimum of physical activity essential for healthy living.

John F. Kennedy

Since former president Kennedy made the above statement, the physical condition of Americans in general has seriously declined. The 2007 article "Dangers of a Sedentary Lifestyle— Disease Risks Associated to Physical Inactivity," by D. E. Stanelli, presented this overview of the current situation:

- In the United States about 300,000 deaths occur annually due to inactivity and poor dietary habits.
- Less active adults are at greater risk of dying of heart disease and developing chronic ailments such as colon cancer, high blood pressure, and type 2 diabetes.
- Nearly 60 million Americans have a form of heart or blood vessel disease.

- 60% of American adults fail to engage in suggested amounts of exercise.

- Older people are commonly less active than younger adults.

- Less affluent individuals tend to be less active than affluent individuals.

- Physically inactive people often have weaker support systems from family and friends.

- Disabled people are less likely than people with no disabilities to engage in moderate physical activity.

- U.S. women tend to be more sedentary than men.

- By age 75, approximately 50% of women and 33% of men partake in no physical activity.[1]

When *National Geographic* took an in-depth look at the secrets of long life in three hotbeds of longevity, they found that the inhabitants of Sardinia, Italy; Okinawa, Japan; and the Seventh Day Adventists in Loma Linda, California, had five practices in common: no smoking; putting family first; staying active; staying socially engaged; and eating many fruits, vegetables, and whole grains.[2]

Researchers have found that even those with chronic health issues such as type 2 diabetes can reduce their chance of developing heart disease by as much as 39 percent through moderate activity and as much as 48 percent by being highly active. "Researchers at the National Public Health Institute in Finland . . . found that people with type 2 diabetes who engaged in moderate or high levels of physical activity were far less likely to die from heart disease than those who engaged in low levels of physical activity. The benefits of physical activity were consistent regardless of body mass index, blood pressure or cholesterol levels or whether or not the person smoked. Benefits were the same in both men and women."[3]

Many seniors love sports and can be found biking or race walking, playing tennis or golf, and even competing in the senior Olympics. But gardening, housecleaning, washing your car, and walking your dog around the block all count, and the positive results accumulate. The important thing is to find something you enjoy and just do it. You'll be healthier and happier and even possibly live longer as a result. In the long term, few things as simple and inexpensive as this return more health benefits. "By age 80, the amount of additional life attributable to adequate exercise, as compared with sedentariness, was one to more than two years."[4]

"When Frank Shearer first put on water skis in 1939, they were wooden planks with rubber straps screwed on top. Now he's 100 years old, far better equipped, and still kicking up the spray near his home in Washington State. 'I like the outdoors and the exercise,' he says. 'And with waterskiing, there is always an extra little charge.'"[5]

You don't have to water-ski or become a mountain climber or marathoner or downhill skier to get the benefits. Moderate exercise for thirty to sixty minutes most days would be a huge advance for most Americans. If you've been living a less-active lifestyle, you should get a physical and then begin with small doses and gradually work your way up. However you start and whatever you do, remember, "There is a fountain of youth. Millions have discovered it—the secret to feeling better and living longer. It is called staying active. You're it. Get fit!"[6]

61

Stay Connected

We cannot live only for ourselves. A thousand fibers connect us with our fellow men.

Herman Melville

All our lives we are encouraged to be independent, strong, and masters of our own destinies. But statistically, "lone rangers" don't live as long, much less as happily, as socially attached people. Remember, even the Lone Ranger had Tonto.

Staying involved often spells the difference between aging gracefully and just growing old. Our total life experience prepares us to share and celebrate life with others, including comforting, teaching, and encouraging those who need it. If we don't share our experience and knowledge, we quickly turn inward and shrivel up emotionally. We gradually become more withdrawn, isolated, and disconnected—a pathway to unhappiness, disease, and early death. Others need you, and you need them.

Researchers have recently found that "a [low] psychological sense of belonging is a greater predictor of major depression than other factors commonly associated with depression, such as social support, conflict, and loneliness."[1]

An Australian longitudinal study related to aging stated "Greater networks with friends were protective against mortality in a ten year followup period."[2]

A study at Wake Forest School of Medicine and Emory University showed that belonging to a club, church, or volunteer group is as health enhancing as beginning exercise or quitting smoking.[3]

Jim's uncle Will was a great example of a life lived to the fullest. Always interested in family, friends, and his community, he never knew a day without purpose and laughter. He learned the joy of gardening from his father and could be found every day of the growing season out among his rows of corn and prize-winning tomatoes. He sent away for historic heirloom seeds and carefully dried the resulting seeds for the next year, so the species would never be lost. A lifelong lover of music, he embraced his talent in multiple ways. As a young man he earned passage to Europe playing his saxophone in the ship's dance band and then toured Europe on his motorcycle, playing with bands along the way. In later years he was always surrounded by the music he loved and sang in his church's choir. Upon retirement he pursued his love of travel and spent many years skipping across the country in his RV bringing his wonderful stories and great sense of humor to everyone he met. He even engaged people as he traveled, flipping on his CB radio and chatting with anyone nearby who would respond.

In his 80s Uncle Will slowed down physically with orthopedic limitations, but his caring heart and love for people became even more of a driving force. He refused to give up his daily walk and inspired many a young athlete as he circled the track using his walker. He was a magnet for all who knew him in the retirement home, encouraging friends and staff alike with his amazing World War II stories of his buddies' courage and triumph. He remained young at heart and socially engaged despite all the changes life had to offer until he died at age 85.

In the creation story, the first thing God pronounced "not good" was a human being alone. We all need both the *feeling* of belonging and the *reality* of belonging. People who stay connected retain a reason to live, long after their "Lone Ranger" counterparts have departed.

There are many ways to get connected, if you're not connected enough already, to those around you. Start first with the healthiest of your social relationships and join with your friends in some of their activities, such as social clubs, a bowling or golf league, some kind of charity work, or a group organized around a hobby. Take a course in something you've always wanted to learn, where it's likely you'll meet others with interests similar to your own. If you have some expertise in an area of interest to others, including those much younger than yourself, become a coach or mentor to one of them, or a group of them, which could give you a whole new view on the world—their world— and even help to make it better.

62

Stay Creative

Stay young by taking inspiration from the young in spirit who remained creatively active all their lives: Goethe completing *Faust* at 80; Titian painting masterpieces at 98; Toscanini conducting at 85; Justice Holmes writing Supreme Court decisions at 90; Edison busy in his laboratory at 84; and Benjamin Franklin helping to frame the American Constitution at 80.

Author unknown

Want to live a long, healthy, productive, and satisfying life? Make something. It doesn't have to be a masterpiece, nor do you have to show it to anybody, because the most positive effect of creativity has nothing to do with other people. It's all about what happens within yourself as you engage your entire self in a creative endeavor.

When you were young, you spent your days playing and making things just using your imagination—sand castles, forts, inhabitants for your dollhouse, finger paintings for your mom, mud pies for your dog, a catnip toy for the cat . . . whatever. But now that you're an adult, that kind of imagination seems to have departed—or has something else happened? Pablo Picasso said, "All children are artists. The problem is how to remain an artist once he grows up."

"As adults we tend to get bogged down in our ideas about ourselves, identifying with past experiences and unconsciously creating limitations," writes Hannah Albert. "To move towards wellness requires holding a vision of where we are going and knowing we deserve to have what we want. Writing, visual art, dance, music and other ways of expressing who we are engages us and assists us in our healing by showing us parts of ourselves we never knew existed."[1]

The first sentence of the Bible is, "In the beginning God created the heavens and the earth" (Gen. 1:1). And when God got around to creating humans, He made us in His own image. Without doubt, the ability to create is one thing that reflects that image, and this is true not only of people named Michelangelo, Mozart, and Tolkien; it is true of you as well.

According to Gene D. Cohen, MD, PhD, lead researcher of a twenty-five-year study on creativity and aging involving more than two hundred senior citizens, "Expressing ourselves creatively can actually improve health, both mentally and physically. Creativity is a natural, vibrant force throughout our lives— a catalyst for growth, excitement and forging a meaningful legacy." Dr. Cohen relates creativity to wellness in a variety of ways:

- Creativity reinforces essential connections between brain cells, including those responsible for memory.
- Creativity strengthens morale. It alters the way we respond to problems and sometimes allows us to transcend them. Keeping a fresh perspective makes us emotionally resilient.
- Challenging the brain can relieve sleep and mood disorders.
- Reading, writing, and word games increase one's working vocabulary and help to fend off forgetfulness.
- Capitalizing on creativity promotes a positive outlook and sense of well-being. That boosts the immune system, which fights disease.
- Having an active, creative life makes it easier to face adversity—including the loss of a spouse.[2]

According to Shaun McNiff, PhD, provost of Endicott College in Beverly, Massachusetts, and a founder of art therapy, which incorporates art and psychotherapy, "you need to commit to being creative in the same way that you need to commit to following a physical fitness routine." He says that "being creative can get endorphins, your body's natural painkillers, going in the same way exercise does, and that once you get into the routine, you begin to crave that endorphin rush much the way you might crave the way exercising makes you feel."[3]

Creativity almost always involves taking a risk and trying something new and not being afraid to fail, or even to succeed. It's about letting go of our fears, discovering new facets of our being, and giving our right brains free reign. Creativity can keep us mentally alert, give us a sense of purpose and meaning, provide us with a way of expressing ourselves, develop our self-esteem and sense of well-being, provide social contact, and reduce isolation and depression, regardless of our circumstances.

The great French Impressionist Pierre-Auguste Renoir suffered from crippling arthritis. On good days, he instructed his assistants to tie him upright in his wheelchair and stabilize the paintbrush in his curled fist, then move the canvas as he directed, since his painting technique had devolved into short jabbing motions forward. When he could no longer sit, he lay in bed and talked an artist through creating the clay sculpture he could see in his mind. His perspective was, "The pain passes, but the beauty remains." He painted a picture the very day he died.

Isn't it time to revisit abandoned passions, even if only to keep your mind functioning efficiently and your dreams alive? What would you like to pass on to your children and grandchildren? Your church might appreciate your ideas for a special project. Family stories will be lost if you don't record them. That one perfect rose might never be seen unless you paint it. The sound of a special composition may be lost for all time if you don't dust off the piano. And remember that gizmo you thought up and vowed to develop when you had more time? Make the time while you still have the time.

63

Supplement Wisely

I used to have a shelf in my kitchen that was dedicated to my row of bottles. And every day I would take some Vitamin A, B-Complex, Vitamin C, Vitamin E, Zinc, selenium, chromium, dolomite, lecithin . . . and others I've forgotten by now. I thought then, 20 and 25 years ago, that I'd better do this because by the year 2000, I'm sure we'll have evidence that either I should have been doing this, or at least I did not do myself any harm. As it turns out, I was wrong on both counts.[1]

Dr. Paul Williams

In 2002, 62 percent of Americans reported that they had used a supplement during the previous twelve months.[2] In 2005, Dave estimated the number of dietary supplements displayed via the relatively meager shelf space in the local grocery store in his small Colorado town (yes, there was only one such store there at the time): in all, there were more than 350 different containers of vitamins, minerals, combinations of vitamins and minerals, herbs, botanicals, and other supplements available. Obviously people are ingesting supplements, especially multivitamin and mineral combinations, since this has been and continues to be the medical "standard of care," despite increasing evidence that many of these supplements have no scientifically discernible effect on either the improvement of health or the prevention of disease.

Reuters News Service reported in 2007: "No studies have yet found that people benefit from taking multivitamin and mineral supplements, and some studies have found that vitamins like A and iron are toxic at high levels. Beta-carotene has been found to increase the risk of lung cancer in smokers." The same article cited research published in May 2007 by the National Cancer Institute that found that "men who exceeded the recommended dose—taking more than seven multivitamins a week—increased the risk of advanced cancer by about 30 percent."[3]

The fact is that no one knows what many of these products are, what they do, and especially how they interact with each other or with prescription medications the buyer might be taking.[4] So beware . . . and be informed, because what you don't know might hurt you—actually, it might kill you, quickly or slowly, depending on what the product in question is, the dosage, and whether you take it in isolation or with other supplements.

Supplement facts and fiction:

Facts:

- More than 30,000 nutritional supplements are available in the United States. In many cases, the purity and concentration of a particular product's nutrient may not match the manufacturer's claims.[5]

- If your diet is rich in a wide variety of ripe, raw vegetables and fruit daily (see http://www.fruitsandveggiesmatter.gov/ for the new recommendations released in 2005) or you are ingesting the micronutrients of the same via some other means such as whole food concentrates, you probably need only a few additional vitamins or minerals such as calcium or omega-3 fatty acids.[6]

- You should not take any manufactured vitamin or mineral in isolation or in megadoses, except with the advice and consent of your physician.[7]

- Some products are not what they claim to be; for example, some anti-aging[8] products claiming to be "human growth hormone" (HGH) are peddled on the Internet. These are not true HGH, or even synthetic HGH, which is available only by prescription.

- Many products claiming to be natural or organic contain mostly synthetic components.

- Despite all claims made by companies that produce supplements with high ORAC (Oxygen Radical Absorbance Capacity) values, which are determined in a lab, there is no evidence that products with extremely high ORAC values are healthful to humans.

Fiction:

- If you can buy a supplement in a natural food store or online, it must be safe.[9]
- You can believe what you read about supplements in "health" magazines. One such magazine markets hundreds of supplements, many supposedly for specific conditions, even though it is illegal to claim that any nutritional supplement treats or cures anything.
- "Thermogenic" products, meal replacement products, and diet shakes can "burn off" fat.
- Cellulite can be effectively treated with pills, creams, or other supplements; none has been shown to have a permanent effect. One of the more humorous claims related to cellulite was made in 2004 by an Italian jean manufacturer, which touted "jean therapy" for cellulite as a result of friction during wear releasing anti-cellulite cream imbedded in the fabric—for a mere $139 per pair.[10]

64

Surround Sound Your Soul

Music is God's best gift to man; the only art of heaven given to earth, the only art of earth we take to heaven.

Walter Savage Lander

Music has the power to lift our spirits; to touch those places in all of us that are hurting; to make us laugh, cry, love more, hate less. It's hard to stay sad and depressed when music is playing. And singing along, even if you can't carry a tune in a bucket, surrounds your soul with sound even more personally.

Neurologist Dr. Oliver Sacks says, "All of us have all sorts of experiences with music: We find ourselves calmed by it, excited by it, mystified by it and often haunted by it. It can lift us out of depression or move us to tears. I need music to start the day and as company when I drive. I need it when I go for swims and runs. I need it, finally, to still my thoughts when I retire, to usher me into the world of dreams."[1]

The older we get, the more music evokes memories. We hear a song from the past and are instantly transported back to a specific time and place. Music can help us recall what has been forgotten by the conscious mind and can help us access feelings from that place and time. Music has been shown to heal—physically, emotionally, relationally, and spiritually. It seems that this human response is innate, perhaps part of the way God made us in His own image. Music can express what spoken words alone cannot express. Music can help us fully experience hurt, anger, fear, grief, sadness, or other difficult emotions that, when bottled up and tightly held on to, hinder our healing.

"Since the beginning of recorded history," says Amitra Cotrell, "music has played a significant role in the healing of our world. Music and healing were communal activities that were natural to everyone. Ancient Greeks said, 'Music is an art imbued with power to penetrate into the very depths of the soul.'"[2] Indeed, Plato wrote, "Music is a moral law. It gives soul to the universe, wings to the mind, flight to the imagination, a charm to sadness, gaiety and life to everything. It is the essence of order and lends to all that is good, just, and beautiful, of which it is the invisible, but nevertheless dazzling, passionate and eternal form."[3]

Daniel Levitin wrote in *This Is Your Brain on Music*, "Music taps into primitive brain structures involved with motivation, reward, and emotion. . . . Music listening and music therapy have been shown to help people overcome a broad range of psychological and physical problems."[4]

One recent study said, "Previous studies have shown that music can improve motivation, elevate mood, and increase feelings of control in older people. The purpose of this randomized clinical trial was to examine the influence of music as a nursing intervention on osteoarthritis pain in elders." The researchers concluded, "Listening to music was an effective nursing intervention for the reduction of chronic osteoarthritis pain in the community-dwelling elders in this study."[5]

Another study of the effect of music on people with terminal illness found, "Quality of life was higher for those subjects receiving music therapy, and their quality of life increased over time as they received more music therapy sessions."[6]

"In my early days of song writing and working in the music industry," Mike said, "I spent quite a lot of time at nursing homes playing for the patients. I clearly remember one woman who was always slumped over in her wheelchair, not really connected with what was going on . . . until I started playing hymns. Then, she lifted her head, sat up in her chair, and sang every word of those songs. When the music was over, she went back into her own world. The staff said that was the only time she ever said anything."

You don't have to play a musical instrument or be able to sing at all to enjoy music. Music crosses the boundary lines of race, socioeconomics, education, politics, and even religion. Music has the ability to reach into those deep recesses in all of us and tap into our emotions. It can take us places emotionally that mere words often can't. Music is, without doubt, *the* universal language.

Music therapist Dr. Deforia Lane said, "Music has the power to move a person between different realities: from a broken body into a soaring spirit, from a broken heart into the connection of shared love, from death into the memory and movement of life. Music has the power to touch the heart of a child with God."

65

Take a Little Wine?

No longer drink water exclusively, but use a little wine for the sake of your stomach and your frequent ailments.

1 Timothy 5:23 NASB

Over 400 scientific studies support some benefit to drinking red wine. However, there are also numerous horrendous outcomes to drinking too much of any type of alcohol. Consuming more than the recommended amount will not only erase the health benefit but increase the risk of such things as liver disease, diabetes, and certain cancers. Experts always caution: If you do not drink alcohol, don't start. But if you do, take just a little red wine.

The meaning of the apostle Paul's advice to Timothy has long been debated among Christians. Exactly what was Paul advising Timothy to do? Some insist that he was referring to unfermented grape juice and not wine as we define it today. Others believe that he was suggesting what amounted to a medical treatment for Timothy's ailments that were possibly caused by drinking contaminated water. It is certainly not our intention to try to settle this debate, since it is all too often clouded by ideology, but to review the science to date related to possible longevity benefits of drinking wine in moderation, and to make some recommendations related to this.

Dave recalls a Christian cardiologist's comment, around 1990, that those who objected to any use of alcohol were going to have to seriously consider the emerging scientific findings related to the possible health value of red wine. More than fifteen years later, if you Google "wine and longevity" you will come up with more than 1.7 million articles online.

One "12-year study, conducted among more than 13,000 men and women ages 30 to 70 who participated in the Copenhagen Heart Study, revealed that those who drank wine daily were much less likely to die during the study period than those who drank beer or liquor or no alcohol at all."[1]

"A number of population studies have revealed that moderate drinkers of red wine have less heart disease than non-drinkers. As a result it has become widely accepted that a glass or two of red wine per day is good for your heart."[2]

It appears that a substance in red wine called resveratrol, an antioxidant, is the primary source of the benefit in question. The other important protective ingredients are called procyanidins. These ingredients have a potent protective effect on blood vessels and have been shown to reduce blood pressure. Resveratrol or procyanidins are not present in significant number in other liquor or white wines. Neither are they present in significant amounts in some of the less-expensive red wines. Research suggests that superior grapes and careful processing preserves the greatest number of antioxidants.

One recent study said, "Participants who drank on average half a glass, or 1.5 ounces, of wine per day, over a long period, had a 40 percent lower rate of all-cause death and a 48 percent lower incidence of cardiovascular death, compared to the non-wine drinkers (white or red was not specified). Researchers said that life expectancy was 3.8 years higher in those men who drank wine compared to those who did not drink alcoholic beverages. Life expectancy of wine users was more than two years longer than users of other alcoholic beverages." [3]

Moderate consumption of alcohol (beer, wine, or spirits) appears to reduce the risk of dementia and Alzheimer's disease. "Researchers studied individuals participating in the Rotterdam Study (7,983 people aged 55 or older) over an average period of six years. Those who consumed one to three drinks of alcohol per day had a significantly lower risk of dementia (including Alzheimer's) than did abstainers." [4]

If you abstain from alcohol for religious or other reasons, there are other ways to gain some of the health benefits reported here. Increasing your intake of foods such as grapes, cranberries, dark chocolate, apples, pomegranates, raspberries, and even peanuts can give you some benefits. Grape juice (the purple kind) contains high levels of flavonoids, as does nonalcoholic red wine. Also, some whole food supplements benefit the heart in similar ways to drinking red wine. [5]

Consuming alcohol of any kind is controversial in some circles, but facts are facts. So here's our bottom line:

- If you don't drink, don't start. Use an alternative method to gain the benefits related to red grapes.
- If you do drink, limit your consumption to two drinks per day for men, one for women, and stick to good quality red wine.
- Do not ignore the calories involved if you are trying to control your weight. Wine can run from 80 to 140 calories per 4-ounce serving; mixed drinks can run much higher. Beer averages nearly 150 per 12 ounces of regular; 110 for "light" beer. So, two drinks of light wine (80 calories) per

day add 58,400 calories to your diet annually. Four ounces of grape juice has about the same effect.

- The annual cost of two glasses of light wine per day would be $672 per year at an average of $1.00 per drink. If taken at a bar, multiply by four to six.

In addition to the above considerations, consequences of alcohol abuse include physical impairment when driving or working, impaired judgment in general, and diminished self-control, sometimes leading to outbursts of anger or physical or sexual abuse. So ask yourself if these things are worth risking in view of the relatively small longevity value of "taking a little wine," when you may be able to obtain similar benefits without consuming alcohol.

66

Take a Nap

You must sleep sometime between lunch and dinner, and no halfway measures. . . . Don't think you will be doing less work because you sleep during the day. . . . You will be able to accomplish more. . . . When the war started, I had to sleep during the day because that was the only way I could cope with my responsibilities.[1]

Winston Churchill

Nap-taking contributes to our general health and well-being, while decreasing the likelihood of accidents resulting from sleepiness. Naps help to short-circuit some of the negative effects on the body arising from chronic sleep deprivation. In fact, napping has even been shown to increase intelligence scores. Taking a "power nap" of fifteen to thirty minutes has the potential of quickly restoring both productivity and positive mood.

"Each year more than fifteen hundred Americans die in an estimated one hundred thousand automobile accidents that are attributed to drowsy driving. Thousands of industrial and other work-related accidents result from drowsiness."[2]

Studies by Dr. Sara Mednick reveal: "Naps have been shown to benefit almost every aspect of human wellness. The benefits to the body include better heart functioning, hormonal maintenance, and cell repair."[3] A large study from the Harvard School of Public Health made startling news in 2007 when it showed that regular nappers were over 30 percent less likely to die of heart disease![4]

Dr. James B. Maas, a psychologist and sleep expert at Cornell University, believes naps should have the same status as daily exercise because of their success in greatly strengthening our ability to make critical decisions and to pay close attention to detail. He promises that short, daily naps are far healthier than sleeping in, taking long weekend naps, or even the caffeine pick-me-up that is powerless to settle our sleep debt.[5]

Dr. William Anthony, professor at Boston University, and his avid-napper wife, Camille, have created a napping advocacy organization and recently designated the first Monday following Daylight Savings Day as National Workplace Napping Day. In their books *The Art of Napping* and *The Art of Napping at Work*, the Anthonys build a logical and watertight case for reviving the practice of napping. They highlight the rich and famous who napped unabashedly, among them presidents, artists, scientists, and generals. "Picture a general napping near the battlefield.

Is this not the ultimate power nap? Napoleon Bonaparte and Stonewall Jackson napped during battles."[6]

In modern-day Washington, President George W. Bush was not a napper, but he nonetheless celebrated the napping prowess of his White House comrades. He created the Annual Brent Scowcroft Award honoring his national security advisor's ability to take power naps. The award was given to "the person who can go to sleep in the most obvious and seemingly embarrassing of all situations without any remorse whatsoever."[7] Mr. Scowcroft, who was in his mid-sixties at the time he held office, greatly benefited from his napping abilities and was able to stay energized and focused despite his intense fourteen-hour days. He was a master napper and could fall asleep anywhere, from the Oval Office to state dinners. He sometimes cleverly masked his downtime by emulating Rodin's sculpture *The Thinker*.

The success of Mr. Scowcroft, and others like him, proves the benefits of napping, as listed by The Sleep Foundation, which claims that napping:

- Restores alertness
- Enhances performance
- Reduces mistakes and accidents
- Promotes relaxation
- Rejuvenates[8]

Lack of rest contributes to problems that can affect all aspects of life. Difficulty concentrating, low energy, pessimism, and irritability are just a few of the many ill effects. Workplace and driving injuries and a number of dangerous medical conditions are associated with lack of sleep, and the answer is not coffee or employing absurd techniques to stay awake or even eyelid toothpicks, but napping, which was what a State Patrol officer "prescribed" for the woman in this true story:

Christian Pruett couldn't believe what he was seeing as he pulled alongside a car that was drifting in and out of a traffic lane on northbound Interstate 25 Monday morning . . . going between 40 to 50 mph. "I honked my horn, but she didn't seem to react at all," Pruett said. . . . That's when he pulled alongside and saw the driver's head leaning back. He called the State Police twice (but they) had no patrol cars close enough to dispatch. Eventually a trooper pulled her over, issued a ticket and told the driver to pull into a parking lot and get some sleep. The State Patrol spokesman later said, "It's not that she was asleep, but she was apparently . . . dozing off."[9]

67

Take a Walk

An early morning walk is a blessing for the whole day.

Henry David Thoreau

Taking a walk can open the door to adventure, play, exercise, spiritual communion, weight loss, stress relief, strengthening friendships, problem solving, or bonding with your spouse or your dog, or both. These are only a few of the many benefits of obeying the old adage "Go take a walk."

Over a twelve-year period, the Honolulu Heart Program studied eight thousand men ages 28 to 62, finding that those who walked just two miles a day cut the risk of dying prematurely by almost 50 percent.[1]

"Walking can reduce the risk of many diseases—from heart attack and stroke to hip fracture and glaucoma. These may sound like claims on a bottle of snake oil, but they're backed by major research. Many other studies indicate a daily brisk walk can help prevent depression, lengthen life span, lower stress levels, relieve arthritis and back pain, strengthen muscles, bones, joints, improve sleep, and elevate mood and sense of well-being."[2]

Walking has even been linked to avoiding gallbladder surgery. Harvard researchers found that in a group of sixty thousand women ages 40 to 65, regular walking or other physical activity lowered the risk of gallbladder surgery by 20 to 31 percent.[3]

Bobbie's mom used to say, "If you're feeling a little down, just take a walk." She lived by the ocean and during the winter, when only the "natives" were there, it could get quite bleak at times. Her cure was to walk along the beach and then into town where she was sure to see a friend or could always buy a piece of fudge for the trip home! Research supports her advice. "A single session of moderate-intensity exercise, such as a thirty-minute walk, improves important mood markers of depression, says a U.S. study of people with major depressive disorder."[4]

We should take a cue from our pets. Our dogs know the world beyond the front gate promises fun and freedom. It's a world of wonder and intrigue filled with sights, sounds, and smells to savor, even if they just walked the same path with us yesterday. They're always ready to chase a squirrel, drink from a stream, tear through the woods to the top of the hill, have a game of chase with their Labrador buddy, play Frisbee with us, or check on that bone they buried yesterday. They're not thinking about the health benefits of getting more exercise, but they surely do get it, and they can help us get it too.

Walking is the ultimate healthy multitasking opportunity.

- Bobbie loves to "prayer walk," and some of her best times have been alone with her God along a beautiful wooded path.[5] You can commune with the Lord or become more aware of the yearnings of your own heart more easily when the cares and chores of the day seem miles away.

- Birdwatchers know the joys of walks along nature trails, anticipating at every turn a chance to see that particular small amazing creature they have been searching out.

- Many avid walkers walk to their favorite music. This combination brings great benefits to their mind as well as to their body and soul.

- Dave and his wife, Ilona, know the deep pleasure of walking through the Rocky Mountain forests near their home in search of wild mushrooms, sharing a world apart that so few get to enjoy, lost in the beauty of God's creation. And sometimes when they take a morning walk near their home with Brownie, their English springer spaniel, they'll encounter a fox, some deer, or even a small herd of majestic elk.

- Grandparents know the fun and surprises encountered as they take adventure walks with their grandchildren.

- Want a sport you can do till you are 95? Take up racewalking. Join Jim and Bobbie and the hordes of walkers who congregate across the country to compete and support worthy causes.

Creativity blossoms and insights increase while you walk. For example, Robert Frost saw two roads diverging in a yellow wood as a metaphor for some of life's more difficult decisions, each of them leading to other choices from which it is usually quite difficult to return. Henry David Thoreau gained inspiration from his walks near Walden Pond. He wrote, "I went to the woods because I wished to live deliberately, to front only the essential facts of life, and see if I could not learn what it had to teach, and not, when I came to die, discover that I had not lived."[6]

These great authors saw things others miss because most people are always rushing and do not train their eyes to really see! Each time we venture outside for a walk we can enrich our lives by really noticing what is there.

Walking is one of the best exercises because it has numerous benefits and almost everyone can do it. It is usually injury free and can be a solo experience or part of a social time with friends or family.

So what are you waiting for? Go take a walk and see what adventures await you!

68

Tune Your Immune

There are conditions under which the most majestic person is obliged to sneeze.

George Eliot

A single sneeze can contain up to forty thousand droplets traveling at one hundred–plus miles per hour for a distance of twelve feet or more. Think of that the next time you're in an elevator and someone who is obviously sick sneezes. When such an event occurs, you wait and you worry and you wonder—*am I going to get that, whatever it was?* Answer: maybe; maybe not. It's primarily up to your immune system.

Have you ever wiped the doorknob of a public bathroom or the handle of the grocery store shopping cart, trying to keep those "germs" away? Here's an estimate of germs *per square inch* on a few surfaces you're likely to encounter: toilet seat: 49; photocopy machine: 69; fax machine: 301; computer mouse: 1,676; office desktop: 20,961; phone receiver: 25,127.[1]

We are surrounded by (and full of) all kinds of pathogens including viruses, bacteria, fungi, protozoa, parasites, cancer cells, toxins, and prions (proteins that cause diseases such as "mad cow disease"). Whether or not these make us sick or even kill us depends on whether or not we have a well-functioning immune system, which is an awesome work of divine art. Research is showing that "immune system cells are connected to each other by an extensive network of tiny tunnels that, like a building's hidden pneumatic tube system, are used to shoot signals to distant cells."[2] When healthy, our immune system is more efficient than the best trained army at eliminating invaders. When unhealthy, we are definitely at risk.

This intricate system has numerous parts:

- Skin and mucous membranes: Unless there is a cut, scrape, or wound, invaders cannot gain access through our skin. Other possible entry points are the nose, mouth, and other body orifices.
- Lymphatic vessels: This is the circulatory system for the immune system. Should an invader gain entrance, there is a quick, aggressive attack.
- White blood cells: There are many types of white blood cells that have specialized and critically important functions. For instance, the T lymphocytes race around and turn various functions on or off. The B lymphocytes manufacture antibodies and the larger phagocytes clean up debris.

The killer cells are on a search-and-destroy mission and move quickly to any invasion site.

- Additional parts of the immune system include the tonsils, adenoids, thymus, spleen, lymph nodes, appendix, and certain areas of the bone marrow.[3]

Many studies warn that chronic stress can decrease immunity and bring on illness or even begin a disease process. Prolonged and extreme grief, for example, depresses T cells. When T cells are altered they can set up an inflammatory response, which can lead to many age-related diseases such as arthrosclerosis, dementia, osteoporosis, and tumors.[4]

Another malfunction allows our immune system police to attack our own body tissues, producing conditions called "autoimmune diseases." These diseases include lupus and rheumatoid arthritis. Recently an astounding discovery was made by Kevin Tracey, MD, "showing that the brain talks directly to the immune system, sending commands that control the body's inflammatory response to infection and autoimmune diseases. Dr. Tracey discovered that the vagus nerve speaks directly to the immune system through a neurochemical called acetylcholine. And stimulating the vagus nerve sent commands to the immune system to stop pumping out toxic inflammatory markers."[5] This important discovery will bring hope to those afflicted with autoimmune diseases.

Boosting our immune systems will never be accomplished by simply swallowing a magic pill or potion, but there are ways to accomplish this naturally. For example, moderate exercise has been shown to boost immunity. Practicing our faith can also improve our immune responses. "A study of 1,700 older North Carolina adults by Duke University found that those who attended church were 50 percent less likely to have blood elevations of IL-6 (a blood protein which indicates an impaired immune system when elevated)."[6] Researchers are beginning to investigate the effects of prayer and meditation on the vagus nerve's role in calming down a high-level inflammatory response.

You do not have to wait until you become ill to know if your immune system is functioning properly. Several blood tests, including the C-reactive protein test, can measure the health of your system. Many physicians are now suggesting this as part of a yearly checkup. Also, the number of colds you get a year provides an idea of how well your army within is functioning. The size and number of lymph glands you are able to see or feel can indicate how well your body is disposing of foreign substances. An excess or enlargement of glands may indicate subpar performance. If you are noticing delayed healing with little cuts or scrapes, check it out with your doctor. Your immune system may need a tune-up.

69

Value Yourself

Until you value yourself, you won't value your time. Until you value your time, you will not do anything with it.

M. Scott Peck, MD

Take a moment and make a list of the five things you value most in life. Are they family, money, material possessions, your job, God, your friends, or something else? Rank these things in order of importance. Are you on your own "most valuable" list? If not, why not?

The word *self-esteem* first appeared in 1657, but by 2003 it had become the third most frequently occurring theme in psychological literature. By then, over twenty-five thousand articles, chapters, and books had referred to the topic, which includes concepts like self-regard, self-respect, self-confidence, and self-worth.[1] The degree to which we esteem ourselves has a significant impact on our choices and actions. If we believe that we have little value, we act as if it doesn't really matter what we do or what the consequences may be. If we believe that we have intrinsic value—value that is not based on things like our looks, our intelligence, or our achievements—then we are more likely to choose friends and activities and to adopt goals consistent with that belief. For example, if a person really believes that he or she is loved unconditionally, then he or she is more likely to engage in constructive behavior, including activities that express positive regard and respect for themselves and others.

Psychologist and self-esteem expert Nathaniel Branden describes self-esteem as "the experience of being competent to cope with the basic challenges of life and being worthy of happiness."[2] He also states that "persons of high self-esteem are not driven to make themselves superior to others, they do not seek to prove their value by measuring themselves against a comparative standard. Their joy is being who they are, not in being better than someone else."[3] Branden labeled external validation as "pseudo self-esteem," arguing that "true self-esteem" comes from internal sources, such as self-responsibility, self-sufficiency, and the knowledge of one's own competence and capability to deal with obstacles and adversity, regardless of what others think. "Positive self-esteem is the immune system of the spirit, helping an individual face life problems and bounce back from adversity."[4]

Jennifer grew up in a family that based its value on physical appearance. Her mother was a former beauty queen who believed her daughter would follow in her footsteps.

My mother signed me up for every beauty pageant around as a young child. . . . As I aged into puberty, I started filling out in ways that were not pleasing to my mother and definitely were not beauty pageant material. I developed anorexia in order to keep my weight down. This unhealthy trend continued until I was hospitalized in my teens due to carrying 100 pounds on my 5′8″ frame. Additional hospitalizations and years of therapy have helped me live a healthier lifestyle. I based my value on what I looked like, partly as a result of what my mother valued. I have since become more aware of who I am, and what I want out of life. After nearly dying because of my disease, I now value making healthy food choices and getting the right amount of exercise.

Jennifer sought approval, something very valuable to her, by trying to keep herself thin, which she believed to be part of looking beautiful, with the result that she became obsessed with that one aspect of herself. But when we properly value ourselves, we will try to become all we were created to be in order to please the One who made us, instead of doing all we are expected to do in order to gain acceptance from the people around us.

Humility is surely a virtue, and pride is the pathway to perdition, but through the years so many have sung the lyrics penned by Isaac Watts, they have internalized them: "Alas! And did my Savior bleed, and did my Sovereign die! Would he devote that sacred head for such a worm as I!" Watts's point was not that we are as valuable as "worms," but that the Lord loved us so much He chose to die for us. This foundational truth of our faith means that God values us very much, and that people of faith should have neither a higher nor a lower value of themselves than does their Redeemer.

When you achieve this perspective, you will take your health more seriously and seek to achieve and maintain optimal health in order to serve your one true Sovereign, not the whims or fancies of those around you or the changing winds of societal norms. Since He loves you, you can value yourself and ignore those who take pride in their humility.

Even if you grew up in the context of "worm theology," you can still change how you perceive and value who you are. Recognize your attributes and celebrate your strengths, rather than dwelling on your weaknesses and imperfections. Have a healthy and positive attitude toward yourself, because you really are here for a reason. People who value themselves tend to have healthier and better relationships, are generally happier, and take care of themselves better, including making better choices in terms of things that affect their health. As author and business philosopher Jim Rohn says, "Take care of your body. It's the only place you have to live." If you were to translate that into spiritual terms, you might say, "I'll take care of myself because Someone bigger than I thinks I am valuable, and I want to serve Him with all my strength, as long as He leaves me here. If my body really is the 'temple of the Holy Spirit,' I'm sure not going to insist on Him living in a dump!"

70

Volunteer and You'll Never Be Bored Again

It is one of the most beautiful compensations of this life that no man can sincerely try to help another without helping himself.

Ralph Waldo Emerson

A volunteer is a person who freely chooses to serve a community or some other cause without being paid for services rendered, though in some cases organizations do reimburse expenses. According to the U.S. Bureau of Labor Statistics, about 61.2 million people volunteered through or for an organization at least once between September 2005 and September 2006—a whopping 26.7 percent of the population! The average time given was just over fifty hours per year. Women volunteered at a higher rate than men across all age groups, educational levels, and other major characteristics. Persons ages 35 to 54 continued to be the most likely to volunteer (31.2 percent), while persons in their early twenties were the least likely (17.8 percent). Older volunteers were more likely to volunteer mainly for religious organizations than were their younger counterparts.

People volunteer for a wide variety of personal reasons, but the health benefits from volunteering suggest that volunteers get back as much or more than they give:

- Volunteer work improves one's sense of well-being by enhancing social support networks. People with strong social support networks have lower premature death rates, less heart disease, enhanced quality of life overall, and fewer health risk factors. Being part of a team focused on the achievement of something good can improve one's feeling of self-worth.

- Volunteering can improve one's appreciation of diversity, through working with or helping others with whom one might otherwise not have much contact.

- Volunteering can reduce heart rates and blood pressure, increase endorphin production, enhance immune systems, and combat social isolation by increasing the opportunity for close interpersonal relationships and strengthening a sense of identity.

- Stress-related health problems improve after performing kind acts. Helping reverses feelings of depression and decreases feelings of hostility and isolation that can cause stress, overeating, ulcers, and so forth. A drop in stress may, for some people, decrease the constriction within the lungs that leads to asthma attacks.

- Helping can enhance feelings of joyfulness, emotional resilience, optimism, confidence, and vigor, and increase one's sense of hope versus helplessness.

- When one is involved with something that is challenging, even an adventure of sorts, a decrease in both the intensity and the awareness of one's own physical pain can occur.

- Volunteering can lead to employment with the agency involved or improve chances of employability elsewhere.

Sharon had put in hundreds of volunteer hours at a small nonprofit ministry in her community over the previous three years, when she heard, "You are the most dedicated and loyal volunteer any organization could have." Because she is passionate about the mission of the organization, and because the work she does closely matches her talents, abilities, and interests, those sacrificial hours have been some of the most enjoyable and self-fulfilling she has ever devoted to volunteer activity. "I have found my niche," she says. "If I knew I had six months to live, I wouldn't change anything about what I'm now doing."

Volunteering provides an opportunity to continue to use your talents, training, and life experiences to help others; as a result you may live a longer and more satisfying life. If you want to volunteer, match your service to your situation. If you still have children at home, volunteer at their school, a youth sports team, or another activity in which your children are involved. If you are in your middle years, or even your retirement years, and your family is gone or fairly independent, look at your talents, abilities, and life experiences and choose something that fits who you are and what you are passionate about. Check out opportunities on the Internet or ask around in your community for organizations with current volunteer needs.

Nonprofits always need volunteers, and there are many worthy organizations no matter where you live. If your spare time is limited, you can help a charitable organization with one-time involvements in specific activities. You might volunteer to help out at the local breast cancer walk, for example, or to staff a nonprofit booth at a local event. These short-term commitments are vitally important to charitable organizations, and at the same time offer you the opportunity to do something for others.

Take care not to allow your volunteering to create stress and possibly lead to burnout if it becomes more demanding than it should be. Pace yourself; give a few hours each week or each month, and not more than you feel you can comfortably give without sacrificing time for your family, friends, and other activities. Have firm boundaries around your time, your energy, and what you will and won't do. But do something. As Eleanor Roosevelt said, "When you cease to make a contribution, you begin to die."

Volunteering, whether you are young or old, can provide a fulfilling way to really live, perhaps for the first time.

What Are You Waiting For?

How many psychiatrists does it take to change a lightbulb? One, but only if the lightbulb really wants to change.

Author unknown

Change is one of the hardest things in life. And when it comes to changing components of our lifestyle, even with the goal of improving our health and longevity, we still find it hard to do what we know we should do and to stop doing things that we like to do but are hurting us.

Our goal in this book has been to provide a reader-friendly overview of what the latest scientific studies and experts in the field have to say about what helps to enhance health and to prevent disease, because the improvement of your health and the health of those you love is important to us. We simply cannot accept (nor should you) the inevitability of the estimate published in 2005 in the *New England Journal of Medicine* that if current trends continue, this generation of children could be the first in two hundred years to have a shorter life expectancy than their parents. In a 2003 report, the World Health Organization predicted that by 2015, 400 *million* people would die of chronic illnesses, most of which are preventable. Unless something changes radically, that number could be an underestimate!

The Best Three Places to Start

According to the World Health Organization's report, the top three modifiable risk factors are unhealthy diet, physical inactivity, and tobacco use. So if you are wondering where to start your program of lifestyle renovation aimed at improving your health and increasing your longevity, these three would be excellent choices. In addition, to help you focus first on some of the more foundational chapters in this book, we have chosen six topics that we think merit special attention, plus one other that governs all the rest—"remember who's in charge of your health."

Remember Who's in Charge of Your Health

Be proactive. Prevention of disease is better than treatment of disease that has already begun. Your doctor can help you identify and make healthy decisions, but your doctor can't control your choices, day by day, moment by moment. And that's the real issue—making healthy versus unhealthy choices. You know the phrase, "one day at a time." Well, in our context we would change that to "one choice at a time." It takes about a month to form a new habit. The foundation of any new habit is a series of choices that differ from your old habitual choices. If you really *believe* that you should make certain changes, and you really *want* to make those changes, you actually *can* make those changes if you take responsibility for them and don't allow anyone or anything to dissuade you.

Eat Well, Be Well

The evidence is clear, and its volume is increasing—a diet rich in a variety of nutrient-dense whole foods (fruits, vegetables, grains, berries, and grapes) enhances health and is an important factor in longevity. As a rule of thumb, if you stick with what God made and avoid, as much as possible, what humans have made, you will eat well and be well.

The USDA's 2005 guidelines raised the recommended daily intake of fruits and vegetables to seven to thirteen, depending on gender, age, and physical activity. All the most significant studies related to diet and longevity published in recent years emphasize the consumption of whole foods and minimize the consumption of meat and dairy products. For someone raised on two eggs, over easy, with hash browns, buttered toast, and bacon or sausage, this particular change can be difficult. But unless you think that you are an exception to the nutritional rules governing longevity, making the necessary changes is well worth considering. Make food your friend. Follow the advice of Hippocrates: "Let food be thy medicine." Oh, and don't forget to drink lots of good, clean water with it.

Stay Active

Most of us need to get more exercise, but, as they say in the South, we're "fixin'" to get more exercise as soon as we can get around to it. Fact 1: Our sedentary lifestyle (combined with our poor eating habits) is killing us slowly. Fact 2: Statistics always seem to be about somebody else. For example, if studies showed that 99 percent of people who get less than thirty minutes of exercise per day will die before age 70, about 99 percent of those considering that statistic would include themselves in the lucky 1 percent to whom the statistics did not apply. Suggestion: Turn off the TV and take your dog, cat, gerbil, or goldfish for a walk. Ride a bike or walk instead of driving, whenever you can. Take the flowerpot off the treadmill and actually use the machine. Everything counts. And you're the counter. Choose something you enjoy, put on your Nikes, and just do it!

Don't Smoke or Hang Out with People Who Do

To the question "Mind if I smoke?" the answer is, "Yes, I do. I mind if you smoke near me or in my house, but most of all I mind if you smoke because you're my friend and I want you around as long as I'm around." Worldwide, smoking kills 400,000 people every year. People who smoke live an average of seven less years than those who do not smoke. Secondhand smoke causes approximately 3,400 lung cancer deaths and 46,000 heart disease deaths in adult nonsmokers in the United States each year. If you do smoke, you should quit. Get help doing so if you need it. Each day after you quit, put the money you saved in a safe place. At $3.00 a pack, two packs per day, kicking this habit will save you over $10,000 in the next five years, enough to _____ (you fill in the blank).

Don't Worry

This may be the age of anxiety, but you don't have to be infected with the worry bug, which causes human beings to pace around in circles, wringing their hands. Of course no one, rich or poor, is exempt from the cares of the world. Everyone has his or her own concerns, from health to bills, to the kids' safety, to what china to use when the neighbors come over for tea and crumpets. Worry can grab you by the throat and strangle you emotionally. The more this happens, the more stress and the less joy you'll have. If you worry enough, life will rush past you day by day until your last worry—specifically, that you're dying—comes true. Get yourself a worry box and put all those concerns inside. At least once a year, sort out and discard the worries that are no longer issues, and leave the rest in there. Follow the example of Mary C. Crowley, who said, "Every evening I turn my worries over to God. He's going to be up all night anyway."

Value Yourself

The greatest commandments, which summarize all the rest (according to Jesus) are to love God with all your heart, soul, mind, and strength, and to love your neighbor *as yourself* (see Mark 12:30–31). If you suffer from inferiority or what we called a "worm mentality," nobody *wants* to be your neighbor, guaranteed. As one anonymous twentieth-century philosopher said, "God don't make no junk." That includes you. You are who you are and that's all you have to be. The fact that you are loved by your Maker gives you value—period, the end. So don't let your parents, teachers, boss, spouse, or anybody else take that away. If you choose to place the same value on yourself as He does, you will take care of yourself so you can serve Him with your whole being, for as long as He leaves you here.

Forgive Yourself

Some people spend much of their adult lives on the "witness stand" in the courtroom of their own mind. They are the accused and the accuser, the jury and the judge. In this particular court, they are perpetually guilty, no matter what the charges, and the sentence is always the same—lifelong sorrow and penitence, with no hope of absolution. Unresolved guilt contributes to insomnia, heart palpitations, heartburn (reflux), high blood pressure, abdominal pain, change in bowel habits, and headaches (including migraines). When your guilt has you imprisoned, it may feel good to feel bad, because somehow you think you're so bad you don't deserve to feel good. By contrast, God's view of your sins is that if you have confessed them to Him, you are forgiven . . . so much so, in fact, that He has forgotten them. Would it not be both wise and faithful to forgive them yourself?

Forgive Others

"To err is human; to forgive is divine." When we forgive someone from our heart, we release *ourselves* from bondage to our own anger, resentment, bitterness, hostility, and desire to get even or make the offender "pay." Carrying a grudge can contribute to high blood pressure, hormone changes linked to heart disease, suppression of the immune system, and possibly even impaired brain function and memory. Letting go of that grudge is a certain route toward better health and longer life. The greatest men have been able to forgive even those intent on killing them. Pope John Paul II visited his would-be assassin in prison and forgave him. Mahatma Gandhi forgave his assassin with his last words. Jesus prayed for His assassins, even as He hung on the cross: "Father, forgive them, for they do not know what they are doing" (Luke 23:34).

Nurture Family Relationships

Would you describe a reunion of your family as a sing-along, a squabble, a dialogue of the deaf, or a gathering of strangers—the younger set biding their time until they have access to their elders' estate? Perhaps a better question, considering how today's families are spread out geographically, might be, "*If* your family could have a family reunion, how do you think it would go?" Well, we hope with lots of hugs and laughter and maybe even some singing 'round the campfire, like it was for many families just a couple generations ago when everyone lived within easy driving distance of each other, and some within shouting distance. Today, family members have to work harder to maintain healthy relationships with each other, yet with free Internet calling, and "web" cameras so you can see each other, regular personal contact is possible even at *any* distance, so you can stay connected and keep the bonds of affection strong.

Love God without Being Religious

The practice of personal faith is central to achieving and maintaining optimal health. In the past few years, hundreds of articles and books have been published affirming that faith is healthy—as long as it is internalized and not just for show. For example, although research shows that regular church attendance is linked to longevity, those who attend church for reasons other than spiritual sustenance, including making politically correct social connections or increasing their business contacts, should not expect any health benefits. As the New Testament says, there is a form of religion, and then there is authentic faith.

In general, religions tend to be exclusive. Over time even sincere movements can degenerate into "denominations" with internal struggles over money and power and public reputations that are uncomplimentary to the God of the Old and New Testaments. As Jesus taught, "God is spirit, and those who worship Him must worship in spirit and truth" (John 4:24 NASB). God greatly desires your love and devotion, in spirit and truth, now and on into eternity. Until then, what are you waiting for?

233

Notes

Chapter 1 Accept Your Mortality

1. William P. Cheshire Jr., MD, "Grey Matters: In the Twilight of Aging, a Twinkle of Hope," *Ethics & Medicine* 24, no. 1 (Spring 2008): 11.

2. Centre for Addiction and Mental Health, "Aging Myths and Facts," http://www.camh.net/Publications/Resources_for_Professionals/Older_Adults/rtoa_aging_myths_facts.html.

3. "Religious Orientation Influences Elderly's Fear of Death," http://www.news-medical.net/?id=17507.

4. Robertson McQuilken, "Let Me Get Home before Dark," as quoted in Crawford Loritts Jr., *Make It Home Before Dark* (Chicago: Moody, 2000), 161–62.

Chapter 2 Attend a Healthy Church

1. R. A. Hummer, R. G. Rogers, C. B. Nam, C. G. Ellison, "Religious Involvement and U.S. Adult Mortality," *Demography* 36, no. 2 (1999): 273–85.

2. W. J. Strawbridge, R. D. Cohen, S. J. Shema, G. A. Kaplan, "Frequent Attendance at Religious Services and Mortality over 28 Years," *American Journal of Public Health* 87, no. 6 (1997): 957–61.

3. See the following report about what the Southern Baptists are doing: For Faith and Family, "Are You a Good Steward of Your Health?" http://faithandfamily.com/article/are-you-a-good-steward-of-your-health.

Chapter 3 Avoid Fad Diets

1. See http://www.aolhealth.com/diet/blood-type-diet/review.

2. See PCC Natural Markets, "Dean Ornish Diet," http://www.pccnatural markets.com/health/Diet/Dean_Ornish_Diet.htm.

3. See http://www.aolhealth.com/diet/zone-diet/review.

Chapter 4 Avoid Infections

1. Neil Osterweil. "Health News: Revenge of the Killer Bugs: Emerging Infectious Diseases," WebMD, www.webmd.com/news/20000426/emerging-infectious-diseases.

2. WebMD, "Methicillin-Resistant Staphylococcus Aureus (MRSA)," http://www.webmd.com/a-to-z-guides/methicillin-resistant-staphylococcus-aureus-mrsa-overview.

3. Daniel J. DeNoon, "Diseases from Animals: A Primer," WebMD, www.webmd.com/a-to-z-guides/features/diseases-from-animals-primer.

4. World Health Organization, "Update on Avian Influenza A (H5N1) Virus Infection in Humans," *New England Journal of Medicine* 358, no. 3 (2008): 261–73.

Chapter 5 Avoid the Debt Trap

1. Jean Lawrence, "Debt Can Be Bad for Your Health," WebMD, http://www.medicinenet.com/script/main/art.asp?articlekey=46186.

2. Federal Reserve Bank of Dallas, "Budget to Save," http://www.dallasfed.org/ca/wealth/pdfs/wealth.pdf.

3. These principles are summarized from a wide range of suggestions in numerous books and on various websites, including Free Money Finance, http://www.freemoneyfinance.com/2005/07/hate_financial_.html.

Chapter 6 Be Content

1. D. D. Danner, D. A. Snowdon, and W. V. Friesen, "Positive Emotions in Early Life and Longevity: Findings from the Nun Study," *Journal of Personality and Social Psychology* 80, no. 5 (2001): 804–13.

Chapter 7 Be Kind to Your GI Tract

1. "Gastrointestinal Disorders," Merck Manual Online Medical Library, www.merck.com/mmpe/sec02.html.

2. M. Camilleri and M. G. Choi, "Irritable Bowel Syndrome," *Alimentary Pharmacology and Therapeutics* 11 (1997): 3–15.

3. For more information on IBS, go to www.aboutIBS.org or www.HelpFor IBS.com.

4. According to Wikipedia, probiotics are dietary supplements containing potentially beneficial bacteria or yeasts. According to the currently adopted definition by FAO/WHO, probiotics are: "Live microorganisms which when

administered in adequate amounts confer a health benefit on the host."
Lactobacillus acidophilus is one of the more common of these. "Probiotic"
means "for life."

Chapter 8 Be Thankful

1. R. A. Emmons and M. E. McCullough, "Counting Blessings Versus
Burdens: An Experimental Investigation of Gratitude and Subjective Well-
Being in Daily Life," *Journal of Personality and Social Psychology* 84, no. 2
(2003): 377–89.

2. Ibid.

3. For more ideas on this, see: Diane Eble, "Abundant Gifts," www.abundant-
gifts.com/benefits_of_gratitude.html.

4. Based on Don Hooser, "Thanksgiving Day," *The Good News*, http://www
.gnmagazine.org/issues/gn31/beingthankful.htm.

Chapter 9 Be Who You Really Are

1. As far as we know, this phrase was coined by Austrian psychiatrist
Alfred Adler (1870–1937).

2. George Ludwig, "Leadership Demands Integrity by Example," Frugal
Marketing.com, http://www.frugalmarketing.com/dtb/integrity-by-example
.shtml.

Chapter 10 Break Bread Together

1. Betty Shimabukuro, "The Family That Eats Together . . . Reaps Benefits
Far Beyond the Simple Pleasure of Sharing a Meal," *Honolulu Star-Bulletin*,
September 22, 2004, http://starbulletin.com/2004/09/22/features/story1
.html.

2. Nancy Gibbs, "The Magic of the Family Meal," *Time*, June 4, 2006. See:
www.time.com/time/magazine/article/0,9171,1200760,00.html.

3. Make Your Own House, http://www.make-my-own-house.com/design-
interior-style.html.

4. John Koshuta, "McDonald's Marketing Focused on Children," Organic
Consumer's Association, http://www.organicconsumers.org/articles/article_
8876.cfm.

5. Gibbs, "The Magic of the Family Meal."

Chapter 11 Breathe Clean Air

1. Quoted at http://www.quotegarden.com/car-free-day.html.

2. Jefferson H. Dickey, MD, "Air Pollution and Primary Care Medicine," Greater
Boston Physicians for Social Responsibity, http://psr.igc.org/nrtb-airpo
l-primcare.htm.

3. P. J. Koken, et al., "Temperature, Air Pollution, and Hospitalization for Cardiovascular Diseases among Elderly People in Denver," *Environmental Health Perspective* 111 (2003): 1312–17.

4. According to the EPA, "The PM-10 standard includes particles with a diameter of 10 micrometers or less (0.0004 inches or one-seventh the width of a human hair). EPA's health-based national air quality standard for PM-10 is 50 µg/m³ (measured as an annual mean) and 150 µg/m³ (measured as a daily concentration). Major concerns for human health from exposure to PM-10 include: effects on breathing and respiratory systems, damage to lung tissue, cancer, and premature death. The elderly, children, and people with chronic lung disease, influenza, or asthma, are especially sensitive to the effects of particulate matter."

5. M. L. Bell, et al., "Ozone and Short-Term Mortality in 95 U.S. Urban Communities, 1987-2000," *JAMA* 292 (2004): 2372–78.

6. Environmental Working Group Memo, "100,000 California Kids Breathe Unhealthy Air at School," June 4, 1997, http://www.ewg.org/files/CaKids.pdf.

7. Ibid.

8. "Cutting Air Pollution Ensures Increased Longevity," *The Lancet*, November 23, 2002, accessed at http://health.allrefer.com/news/newsadmin/printable/php?ID=2408.

Chapter 12 Build Strong Bones

1. From "Arthritis Facts," Arthritis Foundation, http://www.arthritis.org/facts.php.

2. "Osteoarthritis, Your Orthopaedic Connection," American Academy of Orthopaedic Surgeons, http://orthoinfo.aaos.org/topic.cfm?topic=A00227.

3. K. C. Kalunian, "Patient Information: Osteoarthritis Treatment," UpToDate for Patients, http://www.uptodate.com/patients/content/topic.do?topicKey=~VKQnMILErLfEi.

Chapter 13 Create Your Legacy

1. Angus Loten, "Why 80 Is the New 30," Inc.com, November 2007.

2. Fran Howard, "Examine Your Life: A Site for Creating a Legacy," www.examineyourlife.com/aboutus.html.

3. Lee Wise, "Create Your Own Positive Memories Legacy," Working Hard at Making a Lasting Impression on Your World, 2003, http://peopleoffaith.com/leave-a-legacy.htm.

4. See "Creating Legacy," Thrive: Coaching, Consulting, & Training, http://www.allthrive.com/legacy.

Chapter 14 Cry More

1. For more on this, see David Biebel, *If God Is So Good, Why Do I Hurt So Bad?* (1989; repr., Grand Rapids: Baker, 2005).

2. For the full lyrics, see CF Devotionals, http://www.cfdevotionals.org/devpg05/de050714.htm.

3. William Frey, *Crying: The Mystery of Tears* (Minneapolis: Winston Press, 1985).

4. Ashley Montagu, "The Evolution of Weeping," *Science Digest*, November 1981, 32.

5. Jerry Bergman, "The Miracle of Tears," *Creation* 15, no. 4 (September 1993): 16–18.

6. Gregg Levoy, "Tears That Speak," *Psychology Today* (July–August 1988): 8–10.

7. Tom Kovach, "Tear Toxins," *Omni* (December 1982), as quoted by Bergman, "The Miracle of Tears."

8. Dr. Kevin Keough, "Possible Health Benefits of Crying," Helium, www.helium.com/tm/339767/scientific-research-supports-accuracy.

9. Ibid.

10. Montagu, "The Evolution of Weeping," 32.

11. Tom Lutz, *Crying: The Natural and Cultural History of Tears* (New York: Norton, 2001).

12. "Why Can't I Cry?" *Men's Health*, http://www.menshealth.com/cda/article.do?site=MensHealth&channel=guy.wisdom&category=howto.guides&conitem=0c2a99edbbbd201099edbbbd2010cfe793cd____&page=2.

13. Charles Downey, "Toxic Tears: How Crying Keeps You Healthy," Third Age, www.thirdage.com/healthgate/files/14240.html.

Chapter 15 Dance–Or Learn To

1. "Let's Dance to Health," AARP, www.aarp.org/health/fitness/get_motivated/lets_dance_to_health.html.

2. "Dance Your Way to a Better Body," Medical News Today, September 25, 2006, www.medicalnewstoday.com/articles/52560.php.

3. "Dancing Away from Heart Failure," *Harvard Heart Letter* 17, no. 6 (February 2007): 7, http://www.ncbi.nlm.nih.gov/pubmed/17328136.

4. "Dance-Health Benefits," Go for Your Life, www.goforyourlife.vic.gov.au/hav/articles.nsf/pages/Dance_health_benefits.

Chapter 16 Develop Resilience

1. Adapted from "Resilience: Build skills to endure hardship," Mayo Clinic.com, July 18, 2007, http://www.mayoclinic.com/print/resilience/MH00078/METHOD=print.

2. Al Siebert, PhD, "Resilience and Longevity," Resiliency Center, 2000, http://www.resiliencycenter.com/articles/resilong.shtml.

3. "Resilience: Build skills to endure hardship," http://www.mayoclinic .com/print/resilience/MH00078/METHOD=print.

Chapter 17 Discover, Use, and Celebrate Your Talents

1. H. Koivumaa-Honkanen, et al., "Self-Reported Life Satisfaction and 20-Year Mortality in Healthy Finnish Adults," *American Journal of Epidemiology* 152, no. 10 (2000), http://aje.oxfordjournals.org/cgi/content/ full/152/10/983#SEC2.

2. Daniel J. DeNoon, "Early Retirement, Early Death?" WebMD, http://www .webmd.com/healthy-aging/news/20051020/early-retirement-early-death.

Chapter 18 Dodge Cancer

1. From "Cancer Facts & Figures," American Cancer Society, 2008, http:// www.cancer.org/docroot/stt/stt_0.asp.

2. "Cancer Proof Your Life," AOL Body, http://www.body.aol.com/condition-center/breast-cancer/awareness-month/prevent.

3. "National Cancer Institute Fact Sheet," www.cancer.gov/cancertopics/ factsheet/physical-activity-qa/print?page=&keyword=.

4. Regina Sass, "Avocados Can Prevent Oral Cancer, Research Shows," http://www.associatedcontent.com/article/369250/avocados_can_prevent_ oral_cancer_research.html?cat=5.

5. MedicineNet.com, "Stomach Cancer Prevention," www.medicinenet .com/script/main/art.asp?articlekey=57344.

6. "Cancer Proof Your Life."

7. N. Fieshner and A. R. Aiotta, "Prostate Cancer Prevention: Past, Present, and Future," *Cancer* (September 24, 2007).

8. National Cancer Institute, www.cancer.gov.

Chapter 19 Don't Give In to Chronic Disease

1. Senior Net, www.seniornet.org/php/default.php?ClassOrgID=5337&Page ID=5541.

2. Adapted from James May, "Coping with Chronic Illness," The Fathers Network, www.Fathersnetwork.org/page.php?page=647&page=647&SESSION =ab227735c19.

3. C. K. Roberts and R. J. Barnard, "Effects of Exercise and Diet on Chronic Disease," *Journal of Applied Physiology* 98 (2005): 3–30, http://jap.physiology .org/cgi/content/abstract/98/1/3.

4. Write Dave at: DBBV1@AOL.COM.

5. B. H. Wager, B. T. Austin, and M. Von Korff, "Organizing Care for Patients with Chronic Illnesses," *The Milbank Quarterly* 74, no. 4 (1996): 511–44.

6. WebMD.com has trustworthy information and www.seniornet.org has excellent online support groups at their "Health Matters" roundtable.

7. Associated Press, "Even with Chronic Illness, You Can Live to Be 100," MSNBC.com, http://www.msnbc.msn.com/id/23115268/from/ET.

Chapter 20 Don't Smoke or Hang Out with People Who Do

1. "State-Specific Prevalence of Cigarette Smoking Among Adults and Quitting Among Persons Aged 18–35 years—United States, 2006," *Morbidity and Mortality Weekly Report* 56, no. 38 (September 28, 2007): 993–96, www.cdc.gov/MMWR/preview/mmwrhtml/mm5638a2.htm.

2. D. W. Bratzler, W. H. Oehlert, and A. Austelle, "Smoking in the Elderly—It's Never Too Late to Quit." *Journal of Oklahoma State Medical Association* 95, no. 3 (March 2002): 185–91, http://www.ncbi.nlm.nih.gov/pubmed/11921870.

3. P. Cicconetti, et al., "Smoking and Survival in Centenarians," *Recenti Prog Med* 95, no. 4 (April 2004): 187–9, http://www.ncbi.nlm.nih.gov/pubmed/15147062.

4. Adapted from Terry Martin, "Smoking Cessation," About.com, http://quitsmoking.about.com/of/nicotine/a/nicotineeffects.htm.

5. Ibid.

6. Ibid.

7. "Health Effects of Smokeless Tobacco," Council on Scientific Affairs, *JAMA* 255, no. 8 (February 28, 1986): 1038–44, http://jama.ama-assn.org/cgi/content/abstract/255/8/1038.

8. "Do Something: How to Talk to Friends and Family about Smoking," http://www.dosomething.org/tipsheet/how_to_talk_to_friends_and_family_about_smoking.

Chapter 21 Don't Worry, Since It Doesn't Change Anything

1. Jean Twenge, "The Age of Anxiety? Birth Cohort Change in Anxiety and Neuroticism, 1952–1993," *Journal of Personality and Social Psychology* (December 2000), excerpted from: http://www.case.edu/pubaff/univcomm/anxiety.htm.

2. E. A. Holman, R. C. Silver, et al., "Terrorism, Acute Stress, and Cardiovascular Health," http://www.ncbi.nlm.nih.gov/pubmed/18180431 (italics added for emphasis).

Chapter 22 Drink Lots of Clean Water

1. This summary is compiled or excerpted from various sources, including sites like these: http://www.depts.ttu.edu/hospitality/indexmain .php?section=161; http://www.faqs.org/nutrition/Smi-Z/Water.html; http:// pwcworks.com/superhydration.html.

2. "Health Library," Mayo Clinic, http://www.cnn.com/HEALTH/library/ NU/00283.html.

3. Dan Negoianu and Stanley Goldfarb, "Just Add Water," *JASN* Express (*Journal of the American Society of Nephrology*) 19 (2008): 2.

4. "Drinking Water Contaminants," U.S. Environmental Protection Agency —Ground Water and Drinking Water, http://www.epa.gov/safewater/hfacts .html.

5. Ibid.

6. "Probe: Pharmaceuticals in Drinking Water," CBS News, March 10, 2008, http://www.cbsnews.com/stories/2008/03/10/health/main3920454 .shtml?source=RSSattr=HOME _3920454.

7. "Bottled Water," Wikipedia, http://en.wikipedia.org/wiki/Bottled_ water.

8. Ibid.

Chapter 23 Eat Well, Be Well

1. See http://www.mypyramid.gov/; see also: http://www.health.gov/ dietaryguidelines/ for the downloadable report, which is packed with valuable dietary advice.

2. "Dietary Guidelines for Americans—2005," http://www.health.gov/ dietaryguidelines/dga2005/document/html/chapter2.htm.

3. "The Nutrition Source," Harvard School of Public Health, http://www .hsph.harvard.edu/nutritionsource/fruits.html.

4. For information on this alternative, e-mail Dave at: DBBV1@AOL.COM.

Chapter 24 Enjoy a Hobby

1. Maggy Howe, "Hobbies Add Meaning to Our Lives—and May Even Help Us Live Longer," http://www.webmd.com/balance/features/living-passionate-life.

2. Quoted in Peter M. Lopez, "Live Longer: 5 Tips for a Happier and Healthier Life That Don't Include Diet or Exercise," http://hubpages.com/hub/ Live-Longer-5-Health-Tips-That-DO-NOT-Include-Diet-or-Exercise.

3. Ted W. Mills, "A Rosarian Reflects on His Hobby," http://www.millsmix .com/newslett/jan03.html.

4. Bill Malone, "Get into a Hobby: It's Good for You!" Malone Counseling & Consulting Services, http://www.canville.net/malone/getahobby.html.

5. Ibid.

Chapter 25 Enjoy Your Work

1. Reuters Health article citation: *American Journal of Public Health*, November 2007, http://health.asiaone.com/Health/Wellness+%2540+Work/Story/A1Story20071004-28422.html.

2. "U.S. Job Satisfaction Keeps Falling," The Conference Board, http://www.conference-board.org/utilities/pressPrinterFriendly.cfm?press_ID=2582.

3. "A Day Without End," *Psychology Today*, November-December, 1992, http://psychologytoday.com/articles/pto-19921101-000006.html.

Chapter 26 Feast on Fiber

1. See High Fiber Health, http://www.high-fiber-health.com.

2. "Dietary Fiber: An Essential Part of a Healthy Diet," Mayo Clinic Tools for Healthier Lives, www.mayoclinic.com/health/fiber/NU00033.

3. "High Fiber Foods." High Fiber Health.com, www.high-fiber-health.com.

4. "Fiber: Start Roughing It," Harvard School of Public Health, http://www.hsph.harvard.edu/nutritionsource/what-should-you-eat/fiber-full-story/index.html.

5. "Bowel Function & Dietary Fiber," http://www.slrhc.org/healthinfo/dietaryfiber/fibercontentchart.html.

6. "Dietary Fiber: An Essential Part of a Healthy Diet," Mayo Clinic Tools for Healthier Lives, www.mayoclinic.com/health/fiber/NU00033.

Chapter 27 Forgive Others

1. "Forgive and Let Live," Newsweek Health for Life—MSNBC.com, September 27, 2004.

2. H. G. Koenig, M. E. McCullough, D. B. Larson, *Handbook of Religion & Health* (New York: Oxford University Press, 2001), 238–40.

3. Christina Puchalski, "Forgiveness: Spiritual and Medical Implications," *The Yale Journal for Humanities in Medicine*, http://yjhm.yale.edu/archives/spirit2003/forgiveness/cpuchalski.htm.

4. Ibid.

5. Everett L. Worthington Jr., *Dimensions of Forgiveness: Psychological Research and Theological Perspectives* (West Conshohocken, PA: Templeton Foundation Press, 1999).

6. Lewis Smedes, *Choices: Making Right Decisions in a Complex World* (New York: Harper & Row, 1986), 23.

7. Worthington, *Dimensions of Forgiveness*.

Chapter 28 Forgive Yourself

1. Tina Coleman, "Guilty as Charged! Now What?" Aurora Health Care, 2005; quotes June Tangney, PhD, a professor at George Mason University in Fairfax, Virginia, and editor of *Self-Conscious Emotions: The Psychology of Shame, Guilt, Embarrassment and Pride.* See http://www.aurorahealthcare .org/yourhealth/healthgate/getcontent.asp?URLhealthgate=%2214250.html.

2. "Guilt 'Bad for Your Health,'" BBC News Online: Health, http://findarticles .com/p/articles/mi_qn4158/is_20000417/ai_n14300814.

3. Cathleen Henning Fenton, "Your Guide to Panic Disorder," About.com: Panic Disorder, http://panicdisorder.about.com/cs/guilt/a/guilt.htm?p=1.

Chapter 29 Fulfill Your Purpose

1. Excerpted from "Good Health Goes Beyond Diet, Exercise, and Stress," *Medical Research News*, August 2004, www.news-medical.net/?id=4074.

2. This fictionalized dialogue is based on a true story.

Chapter 30 Get a Good Night's Sleep

1. S. R. Patel, N. T. Ayas, M. R. Malhotra, et al., "A Prospective Study of Sleep Duration and Mortality Risk in Women," *Sleep* 27, no. 3 (May 1, 2004): 440–44.

2. Jeanie Lerche Davis, "The Toll of Sleep Loss in America," Sleep Disorders Guide, www.webmd.com/sleep-disorders/guide/toll-of-sleep-loss-in-america ?page=2.

3. Ibid.

4. Excerpted from "The Story of Mike H," *The Apnea Patients News*, Education Awareness Network, www.apneanet.org/stories/storymikeh .htm.

Chapter 31 Get and Keep Your Affairs in Order

1. "57% of Americans Do Not Have a Will," BankRate.com, http://investor .bankrate.com/releasedetail.cfm?ReleaseID=276290.

2. "Getting Your Affairs in Order," *Aging and Geriatrics*, National Institute on Aging, www.mentalhelp.net/poc/view_doc.php?type=doc& id=3274&cn=12.

Chapter 32 Get Out There

1. Joan Raymond, "Happy Trails: America's Affinity for the Great Outdoors," from American Demographics, August 2000, accessed at http://findarticles .com/p/articles/mi_m4021/is_2000_August/ai_65300670.

2. "Outdoor Recreation in America," http://www.funoutdoors.com/taxonomy/view/or/62.

3. "Television and Health," The Sourcebook for Teaching Science, http://www.csun.edu/science/health/docs/ tv&health.html.

4. Ibid.

Chapter 33 Hang Loose or Stress Could Get You

1. Bobbie Dill, BSN, RN, et al., "The Registered Nurse's Role in the Office Treatment of Patients with Histories of Abuse," *Gastroenterology Nursing* 20, no. 5 (1997): 162–67.

2. Hans Selye, *The Stress of Life*, 2nd ed. (New York: McGraw Hill, 1978), xv.

3. K. S. Dunn, A. L. Horgas, "The Prevalence of Prayer as a Spiritual Self-care Modality in Elders," *Journal of Holistic Nursing* 18, no. 4 (December 2000): 337–51, quoted in "Prayer Used for Stress," *Star Tribune*, January 13, 2001, B10.

Chapter 34 Have at Least One Close Friend

1. Sharon O'Brien, "Friends are more important than family for longevity," Your Guide to Senior Living, http://seniorliving.about.com/od/lifetransitionsaging/a/longevity.htm.

2. E. Guilley et al., "Association Between Social Relationships and Survival of Swiss Octogenarians," *Aging Clinical and Experimental Research* 17, no. 5 (October 2005): 419–25.

3. Henry Cloud, *Changes That Heal* (Grand Rapids: Zondervan, 1992), 64.

4. Henri J. M. Nouwen, *Out of Solitude: Three Meditations on the Christian Life*, rev. ed. (Notre Dame: Ave Maria Press, 2005), 38.

Chapter 35 Hold On to Hope

1. Viktor Frankl, MD, *Man's Search for Meaning* (New York: Washington Square Press, 1985), 60.

2. Jerome Groopman, MD, *The Anatomy of Hope* (New York: Random House, 2004), xiv.

3. Jamie Shane, "Feeling Unsatisfied? Creating Expectations Only Borrows Trouble," Naples *Daily News*, July 19, 2007, http://www.naplesnews.com/news/2007/jul/19/feeling_unsatisfied_creating_expectations_only_bor.

4. Martin Seligman, "Forum on Depression," *Life Matters*, 2002, http://www.abc.net.au/rn/talks/lm/stories/s648530.htm.

5. James A. Avery, MD, "The 'H' in Hospice Stands for Hope," *Today's Christian Doctor* 34, no. 2 (Summer 2003): 24.

Chapter 36 Keep an Eye on Your Eyes

1. Miranda Hitti, "Many Adults Fuzzy on Eye Health," WebMD Medical News, October 2007, www.webmd.com/eye-health/news/20071019/many-adults-fuzzy-on-eye-health.

2. "14 Million Americans Are Visually Impaired," News-Medical.net, May12, 2006, www.news-medical.net/print_article.asp?id=17936.

3. Email Dave for information on this option: DBBV1@AOL.COM.

4. "Lutein: The Eyes Have It," New Hope, http://www.newhope.com/nutritionsciencenews/NSN_backs/Nov_00/lutein.cfm.

Chapter 37 Keep Your Heart Smart

1. Nursery rhyme quoted by Wayne Fields, *What the River Knows*, 1990.

2. Jeanie Lerche Davis, "Lessons Learned from the Earth's Elders," WebMD with AOL Health, http://aolsvc.health.webmd.aol.com/content/article/113/110882.htm?printing=true.

3. Reported in *JAMA* 296 (1996): 1809.

4. "Depression Raises Heart Risks," *American Journal of Preventative Medicine*, Scout News LLC, http://www.hearttalklive.com/previous.news.php?fWeek=2005-12-25.

5. See http://www.gotohealth.com/showNewsletter.cfm?rec=41.

6. For more information on this option email Dave at: DBBV1@AOL.COM.

Chapter 38 Keep Your Mind Sharp

1. William P. Cheshire Jr., "In the Twilight of Aging, a Twinkle of Hope," *Ethics & Medicine* 24, no. 1 (2008): 9–14.

2. H. B. Lee et al., "Level of Cognitive Impairment Predicts Mortality and High Risk Community Samples: The Memory and Medical Care Study," *Journal of Neuropsychiatry and Clinical Neurosciences* 18 (2006): 543–46, http://neuro.psychiatryonline.org/cgi/content/abstract/18/4/543.

3. "Preventing and Treating Alzheimer's: Prevention, Treatment, and Slowing down the Process," Help Guide.org, http://www.helpguide.org/elder/alzheimers_prevention_slowing_down_treatment.htm.

Chapter 39 Keep Your "Wow" Working

1. Robert J. Campbell, "Dream Stealers, Dream Makers" (sermon, Church of the Covenant, August 27, 2006), http://www.covenantweb.org/sermons/082706.html.

2. Ibid.

3. Rachel Carlson, *The Sense of Wonder* (New York: HarperCollins: 1998), 41.

4. Monte Swan with David Biebel, *Romancing Your Child's Heart* (Sisters, OR: Multnomah, 2002), 219.

5. Isaac Newton, Quotes DB.com, http://www.quotedb.com/quotes/ 3627.

Chapter 40 Know the Skinny on Fat

1. Dariush Mozaffarian, MD, et al., "Trans Fatty Acids and Cardiovascular Disease," *New England Journal of Medicine* (April 13, 2006): 1606, http:// content.nejm.org/cgi/content/short/354/15/1601.

2. Sally Squires, "The Governor Is a Happy Loser," *Washington Post*, August 10, 2004.

3. Ibid.

Chapter 41 Laugh More

1. Marilyn Elias, "A Laugh a Day May Help Keep Death Further Away," *USA Today*, http://findarticles.com/p/articles/mi_kmusa/is_200703/ai_ n18696726.

2. Holistic Online, www.holisticonline.com/Humor_Therapy/humor _therapy_benefits.

3. Larry Wilde, "Up Your Laugh Quotient," http://www.larrywilde.com/ lzone.htm.

4. Proverbs 15:15 NASB; Proverbs 17:22 KJV.

5. P. Spitzer, "The Clown Doctors," http://www.e-bility.com/articles/clown doctors.php.

6. "UAMS Physician Mixes Humor with Good Medicine," UAMS In the News, http://www.uams.edu/update/absolutenm/templates/news2003v2 .asp?articleid=4942&zoneid=18.

7. Wilde, "Up Your Laugh Quotient."

Chapter 42 Lighten Up

1. "Higher and more prolonged levels of cortisol in the bloodstream (like those associated with chronic stress) have been shown to have negative effects, such as: impaired cognitive performance, suppressed thyroid function, blood sugar imbalances such as hyperglycemia, decreased bone density, decrease in muscle tissue, higher blood pressure, lowered immunity and inflammatory responses in the body, as well as other health consequences, increased abdominal fat, which is associated with a greater amount of health problems than fat deposited in other areas of the body. Some of the health problems associated with increased stomach fat are heart attacks, strokes, the development of higher levels of 'bad' cholesterol (LDL) and lower levels of

'good' cholesterol (HDL), which can lead to other health problems!" (http://stress.about.com/od/stresshealth/a/cortisol.htm).

2. Miranda Hitti, "Why Perfectionism Isn't Perfect," WebMD.com, http://www.webmd.com/balance/news/20070504/why-perfectionism-isnt-perfect.

3. Excerpted from "Life Dance," *Today's Christian Doctor* 39, no. 1 (Spring 2008): 18–20.

Chapter 43 Live in the Now

1. From *Ferris Bueller's Day Off*, a 1986 comedy film by Paramount Pictures starring Matthew Broderick, Alan Ruck, Mia Sara, Jeffrey Jones, and Jennifer Grey.

2. Christina Diaz, "What Do You Mean I'm Not Living in the Present?" The Benefits of Positive Thinking, http://www.the-benefits-of-positive-thinking.com/living-in-the-present.html.

3. Michael McGrath, "Learn to Live in the Present with Personal Development," http://www.articlesbase.com/print/313072.

4. Jarrett Bell, "Tragedy Forces Dungy 'to Live in the Present,'" *USA Today*, http://www.usatoday.com/sports/football/nfl/colts/2006-08-31-dungy-cover_x.htm.

5. "Henry David Thoreau (1817–1862) Quotes." http://www.phnet.fi/public/mamaa1/thoreau.htm.

Chapter 44 Love and Be Loved

1. Ann Landers, QuoteWorld.com, http://www.quoteworld.org/quotes/8018.

2. "Healthy Marriage: Why Love Is Good for You," Mayo Clinic, http://www.cnn.com/HEALTH/library/MH/00108.html.

3. M. Langon, "The Health Benefits of Love—How Love Can Improve Your Health," Associated Content, November 13, 2007, http://www.associatedcontent.com/article/443851/the_health_benefits_of_love.html.

4. Ibid.

5. Ibid.

Chapter 45 Love God without Being Religious

1. Jeanie Lerche Davis, "The Science of Good Deeds," WebMD Feature, http://aolsvc.health.webmd.aol.com/content/Article/115/111985.htm.

2. Ervin Shaw, MD, homepage, "Faith Allows Enhancement of Health Status," www.theeffectivetruth.info/fahealth.html.

Chapter 46 Love Your Liver

1. "Facts at a Glance: The Liver and Liver Disease," American Liver Foundation, http://www.liverfoundation.org.

2. "Liver Disease," University of Illinois Medical Center, http://uimc .discoveryhospital.com/main.php?id=3307.

3. "Liver Problems," Mayo Clinic Tools for Healthier Lives, http://www .mayoclinic.com/health/liver/DG00038.

Chapter 47 Mind Your Mouth

1. "Down in the Mouth: Oral Health and the Whole Body," *Fact of Life; Issue Briefings for Health Reporters* 7, no. 5 (May 2002), Center for the Advancement of Health, www.cfah.org/factsoflife/vol7no5.cfm.

2. For more information on this factor, contact Dave at: DBBV1@AOL .COM.

3. R. Rautemaa, A. Lauhio, M. P. Cullinan, and G. J. Seymour, "Oral Infections and Systemic Disease: An Emerging Problem in Medicine," *Clinical Microbiology & Infection* 13, no. 11 (November 2007): 1041–47.

4. Academy of General Dentistry, "Why Is Oral Health Important for Men?" *Oral Health Resources: Men's Oral Health*, March 30, 2007, www.agd .org/support/articles?ArtID=1266.

5. Center for Advancement of Health, "Down in the Mouth: Oral Health and the Whole Body," *Facts of Life: Issue Briefings for Health Reporters.* 7, no 5 (May 2002).

6. Academy of General Dentistry, "Why Is Oral Health Important?"

7. Academy of General Dentistry, "Down in the Mouth."

Chapter 48 Nurture Family Relationships

1. Laura L. Carstensen and Christine R. Hartel, eds., *When I'm 64*, Committee on Aging Frontiers in Social Psychology, Personality, and Adult Developmental Psychology, National Research Council of the National Academies (Washington, D.C.: National Academies Press), 25–26.

2. Les B. Whitbeck, Danny R. Hoyt, and Shirley M. Huck, "Family Relationship History, Contemporary Parent-Grandparent Relationship Quality, and the Grandparent-Grandchild Relationship," *Journal of Marriage and Family* 55 (November 1993): 1025–35.

3. V. Bedford, "Sibling Relationships in Middle Adulthood and Old Age," quoted in R. M. Blieszner and V. H. Bedford, eds., *Handbook on Aging and the Family* (Westport: Greenwood, 1997), 201–22.

4. Frederic M. Hudson, "Mastering the Art of Longevity," from *The Adult Years: Mastering the Art of Self-Renewal* (San Francisco: Jossey-Bass, 1999), http://www.grandtimes.com/Master_Art.html.

5. V. G. Cicirelli, *Sibling Relationships Across the Life Span*, (New York: Plenum Press, 1995).

6. D. Gold, "Sibling Relationships in Old Age: A Typology," *International Journal of Aging and Human Development* 28, no. 1 (1989): 37–51.

Chapter 49 Nurture Something

1. Harvard Vanguard Medical Associates, "Gardening Provides Many Health Benefits," 2007, see: http://www.harvardvanguard.org/info/news/mind/GStone_mb_0607.asp.

2. Karen York, "Grow Better, Feel Better, Garden Longer," http://www.gardenforever.com/pages/artYork.htm.

Chapter 50 Pay the Kindness Forward

1. "Mother Teresa Quotes," BrainyQuote.com, http://www.brainyquote.com/quotes/authors/m/mother_teresa.html.

2. Allan Luks with Peggy Payne, *The Healing Power of Doing Good* (New York: Fawcett, 1991), 87.

3. Gift of Kindness, www.giftofkindness.com.

Chapter 51 Play More

1. Quoted in Dr. Norman Cousins, "Playing Together for Fun: Creative Play and Lifelong Games," HelpGuide.org, February 10, 2007, http://www.helpguide.org/life/creative_play_fun_games.htm.

2. Marianne St. Clair, "The Top 10 Benefits of Play," November 28, 2006, http://www.mariannestclair.com.

3. Cousins, "Playing Together for Fun."

4. "Leisure activities and the risk of dementia in the elderly," *New England Journal of Medicine* 348, no. 25 (June 2003): 2508–16.

5. ThinkExist.com, http://thinkexist.com/quotes/with/keyword/notable.

Chapter 52 Practice Generosity

1. Luks and Payne, *The Healing Power of Doing Good*, 82–83.

2. "Empathy and Oxytocin Lead to Greater Generosity," *Science Daily*, November 8, 2007, www.sciencedaily.com/releases/2007/11/071107074321.htm.

3. "Thinking about God Leads to Generosity, Study Suggests," *Science Daily*, August 31, 2007, www.sciencedaily.com/releases/2007/08/070829102048.htm.

4. Stephen Post, PhD, and Jill Neimark, *Why Good Things Happen to Good People* (New York: Broadway Books, 2007), 2.

Chapter 53 Practice Safe Sex

1. News-Medical.Net. "'Sexercise' Will Keep You Healthy," February 12, 2006, http://www.news-medical.net/?id=15844.

2. News-Medical.Net, "Sex Among Seniors," August 26, 2007, http://www.news-medical.net/?id=29068.

3. "Survey Shows Sexual Health Important Component of Overall Well-Being for Midlife and Beyond," Medical Studies/Trials, May 30, 2005, www.news-medical.net.

4. "Baby Boomers, Sex and HIV," Life Two, November 2007, http://lifetwo.com/production/node/20071126-baby-boomers-and-hiv.

5. "Sexually Transmitted Diseases Fact Sheets," Centers for Disease Control and Prevention, http://www.cdc.gov/STD/HealthComm/fact_sheets.htm.

6. Avis Yarbrough, "STDs and AIDS in Senior Citizens: Does Grandpa or Grandma Have a Venereal Disease?" http://www.associatedcontent.com/article/77843/stds_and_aids_in_senior_citizens.html?cat=5.

Chapter 54 Pray 24/7

1. Marty Sullivan, MD, "The Proven Health Benefits of Spirituality and Prayer," Heart Lung Transplant Support Group, Duke University, http://groups.msn.com/HeartLungTransplantSupportGroup/benefitsofprayer.msnw.

2. Clem Boyd, "The Health Benefits of Prayer," http://iluv2prshim.wordpress.com/2008/03/14/the-health-benefits-of-prayer.

3. Used by permission.

Chapter 55 Prevent Accidents

1. "Accidental Deaths Increasing at Alarming Rate . . ." National Safety Council Press release, www.csrwire.com/PressReleasePrint.php?id=9709.

2. Ibid.

3. Ibid.

4. "Blogs-Safety," *Consumer Reports*, http://blogs.consumerreports.org/safety/2007/09/accidental-deat.html.

5. "Water Related Injuries Fact Sheet," Centers for Disease Control, http://www.cdc.gov/ncipc/factsheets/drown.htm.

6. "Blogs-Safety."

7. "Accidental Death Rate Creeping Higher in U.S.," Associated Press, June 7, 2007, http://www.msnbc.msn.com/id/19080118.

Chapter 56 Remember Who's in Charge of Your Health

1. Russell Wild, "Your Take-Charge Guide to Affordable Health Care," *AARP Magazine*, July/August 2006, www.aarpmagazine.org/health/affordable_health_care.html.

2. Mary Jo Kreitzer, "Taking Charge of Your Health," University of Minnesota, http://takingcharge.csh.umn.edu/healthcare_system.

3. Wild, "Your Take-Charge Guide to Affordable Health Care."

Chapter 58 Seek Solitude

1. Miranda Hitti, "Loneliness May Affect Genes: Certain Genes May Be More or Less Active in Lonely People, Raising Health Risks," WebMD Medical News, September 13, 2007, see http://www.webmd.com/balance/news/20070913/loneliness-may-affect-genes.

2. Christopher R. Long, and James R. Averill, "Solitude: An Exploration of Benefits of Being Alone," *Journal for the Theory of Social Behaviour* 33, no. 1 (2003): 21–44.

3. Fred Smith Sr., "My Friend Fenelon," from *The Pastor's Soul Volume 5: Leading with Integrity*, see http://ctlibrary.com/lebooks/thepastorssoul/soulintegrity/pstsoul5-2.html.

Chapter 59 Simplify Your Life

1. Richard Swenson, *The Overload Syndrome* (Colorado Springs: NavPress, 1998), 11–15.

2. Richard Swenson, *Margin* (Colorado Springs: NavPress, 1992), 206.

Chapter 60 Stay Active

1. D. E. Stanelli, "Dangers of a Sedentary Lifestyle," Suite101.com, http://fitness.suite101.com/article.cfm/deadly_cost_of_physical_inactivity.

2. Dan Buettner, "The Secrets of Long Life," *National Geographic*, November 2005, 2–26.

3. To examine the results of the Finnish study, see "Physical Activity in the Prevention of Type 2 Diabetes," http://diabetes.diabetesjournals.org/cgi/content/full/54/1/158.

4. R. S. Paffenbarger Jr., et al., "Physical Activity, All-Cause Mortality, and Longevity of College Alumni," *New England Journal of Medicine* 314, no. 10 (March 1986): 605–13, http://www.ncbi.nlm.nih.gov/pubmed/3945246.

5. Buettner, "The Secrets of Long Life."

6. "Getting Started!" The President's Challenge, www.presidentschallenge.org/home_seniors.aspx.

Chapter 61 Stay Connected

1. Amy Reyes, "Low Sense of Belonging Is a Predictor of Depression," *Science Daily*, http://www.sciencedaily.com/releases/1999/08/990810164724.htm.

2. L. C. Giles et al., "Effects of Social Networks in Very Old Australians: The Australian Longitudinal Study of Aging," *Journal of Epidemiology and Community Health* 59, no. 7 (July 2005): 574–79.

3. "Belonging to a Club, Church, or Charity as Good for Health as Quitting Smoking or Doing Exercise," *Medical News Today*, http://www.medical newstoday.com/articles/7819.php.

Chapter 62 Stay Creative

1. Hannah Albert, "My Philosophy on Health and Creativity," Fertile Ground, http://www.hannahalbertnd.com/html/philosophy.shtml.

2. Excerpted from Gene D. Cohen, *Welcome to the Creative Age* (New York: Harper, 2001), reviewed at: http://www.demko.com/cb000411.htm.

3. Kathryn Perrotti Leavitt, "Create a Healthy You," BNet.com, http://findarticles.com/p/articles/mi_m0NAH/is_5_32/ai_87854528/pg_2.

Chapter 63 Supplement Wisely

1. Dr. Paul Williams, "In Case of Emergency," audio CD, National Safety Associates, Inc., 2004. For a free copy of this talk email Dave Biebel at DBBV1@AOL.COM.

2. See http://www.newstarget.com/z003557.html.

3. Julie Steenhuysen, "Vitamin Overuse Tied to Men's Cancer Risk," Reuters, May 16, 2007, http://www.boston.com/news/nation/articles/2007/05/16/vitamin_overuse_tied_to_mens_cancer_risk.

4. The most reliable review of herbal remedies, vitamins, and dietary supplements that we know of from a Christian perspective can be found in Donal O'Mathuna, PhD, and Walt Larimore, MD, *Alternative Medicine: The Christian Handbook* (Grand Rapids: Zondervan, 2001), 288–465.

5. You can stay abreast of supplement facts at www.naturaldatabase .com—annual subscription required. The Mayo Clinic's website has free data available on about one hundred supplements. Go to: www.mayoclinic .com/findinformation/druginformation and enter the substance's name. A searchable database is available at: www.cochrane.org. When evaluating any specific product, look for the stamp of approval—USP Verified—of the United States Pharmacopeia (USP): see www.uspverified.org. NSF International maintains a list of supplements that contain what is listed on the label, what is free of contaminants, and what is manufactured in a legitimate way. Or, if you prefer a more lay-oriented but trustworthy evaluation of a variety of supplements, see *Oprah* magazine, June 2004, "A Dose of Reality."

6. Ibid.

7. Reason: Certain common supplements when taken in megadoses or in isolation can have detrimental health effects. These include vitamin E, see http://www.nytimes.com/2004/11/14/opinion/14sun2.html?oref=login;

vitamin C, see http://altmedangel.com/arteries.htm; beta-carotene, see http://www.consumerreports.org/cro/health-fitness/is-a-multivitamin-enough-too-much-1004/index.htm?resultPageIndex=1&resultIndex=5&searchTerm=bet a%20carotene; and iron, which is unnecessary in most people who are eating enough iron-rich foods and can be dangerous, see http://www.bloodbook.com/iron-foods.html.

8. The most effective anti-aging strategy is to reduce oxidative damage to your DNA through ingestion of ripe vegetables; grains; berries, grapes, and other fruits. Since your DNA can only replicate itself about fifty times in your lifetime, the healthier you keep your DNA, the slower you will age.

9. ConsumerReports.org lists the following as the dirty dozen of supplements to avoid: aristolochic acid, comfrey, androstenedione, chaparral, germander, kava, bitter orange, organ/glandular extracts, lobelia, pennyroyal oil, scullcap, yohimbe, see http://www.consumerreports.org/cro/cu-press-room/pressroom/archive/2004/05/eng0405die.htm?resultPageIndex=1&resultIndex=1&searchTerm=dirty%20dozen%20supplements.

10. For more information, see http://healthsearch.aol.com/search?q1=anti-cellulite+cream+jeans.

Chapter 64 Surround Sound Your Soul

1. Oliver Sacks, MD, "When Music Heals," *Parade* magazine, March 31, 2002.

2. Amrita Cottrell, "Healing Music—A Closer Look," The Healing Music Organization, 2000, www.healingmusic.org.

3. Amitra Cottrell, "The Rose of Music and Sound in Healing from Cancer," http://www.healingmusic.org/Library/Articles/MusicAndSoundIn HealingFromCancer.asp.

4. Daniel J. Levitin, *This Is Your Brain on Music* (New York: Plume, 2007), 191, 227.

5. R. McCaffrey and E. Freeman, "Effect of Music on Chronic Osteoarthritis Pain in Older People," *Journal of Advanced Nursing* 44, no. 5 (2003): 517–24.

6. R. E. Hilliard, "The Effects of Music Therapy on the Quality and Length of Life of People Diagnosed with Terminal Cancer," *Journal of Music Therapy* 40, no. 2 (2003): 113–37.

Chapter 65 Take a Little Wine?

1. Jane E. Brody, "Danish Study Shows Wine Aiding Longevity," *New York Times*, http://query.nytimes.com/gst/fullpage.html?res=990CE7D81238F936A35 756C0A963958260.

2. Queen Mary University of London, "Real Link between Drinking Red Wine and Increased Longevity," Home: Food and Health, www.emaxhealth.com/74/8441.html.

3. "Light Wine Intake Is Associated with Longer Life Expectancy in Men," American Heart Association, March 2007, www.supercentenarian.com/archive/wine.html.

4. A. Ruitenberg et al., "Alcohol Consumption and Risk of Dementia: The Rotterdam Study," *The Lancet* 359, no. 9303 (2002): 281–86.

5. For more information on such supplements, e-mail: DBBV1@AOL .COM.

Chapter 66 Take a Nap

1. See http://a.wholelottanothing.org/2007/02/14/1946-action-this-day-the-churchill-centre.

2. David B. Biebel and Harold George Koenig, *Simple Health* (Lake Mary, FL: Siloam, 2005), 53.

3. Sara Mednick, "What Are the Benefits of a Nap?" FAQs about Power Naps, http://www.metronaps.com/mn/studies_resources/faq_about_power _naps.

4. Rob Stein, "Midday Naps Found to Help Fend off Heart Disease," http://www.washingtonpost.com/wp-dyn/content/article/2007/02/12/AR2007021 200626.html.

5. Jane E. Brody, "New Respect for the Nap, a Pause That Refreshes," http://www.physics.ohio-state.edu/~wilkins/writing/Resources/essays/nap_refreshs .html.

6. William Anthony, *The Art of Napping* (New York: Paul Brunton Philosophic Foundation by Larson Publications, 1997), 53.

7. Maureen Dowd, "Remorseless Dozing Gets Presidential Nod," *The New York Times*, May 8, 2006, http://query.nytimes.com/gst/fullpage.html?res=950D E7DF1F3CF933A25752C1A96F948260.

8. "The Short Story on Napping," http://www.sleepfoundation.org/site/c .huIXKjM0IxF/b.2419153/k.8430/The_Short_Story_on_Napping.htm.

9. John C. Ensslin, "Caught on Tape: Dozy Driver Swerves 30-Plus Miles on I-25. Witness Questions Patrol's Response Time to Incident," *Rocky Mountain News*, October 18, 2007.

Chapter 67 Take a Walk

1. A. A. Hakim et al., "Effects of Walking Among Nonsmoking Retired Men," *New England Journal of Medicine* 338 (1998): 94–99.

2. "Walking: The Numerous Benefits of Walking," AARP, www.aarp.org/health/fitness/walking/a2004-06-17-walking-numerousbenefits.html.

3. Ibid.

4. "Moderate Exercise Boosts Depressed People," Health Scout, Scout NewsLLC, 2006, see www.heartinfo.org.

5. For more information about "prayer walking" and its benefits, see Janet Holm McHenry, *PrayerWalk* (Colorado Springs: WaterBrook, 2001).

6. Henry David Thoreau, *Walden* (1854).

Chapter 68 Tune Your Immune

1. Ronald Klatz and Robert Goldman, *Infection Protection: Pandemic* (Chicago: American Academy of Anti-Aging Medicine, 2006).

2. News-Medical.Net, "Surprising Immune System Cells Discovery," *Medical Research News*, September 26, 2005, see http://www.news-medical .net/?id=13316.

3. Ibid.

4. A. Burkle et al., "Pathophysiology of Ageing, Longevity and Age Related Diseases," *Immunity and Ageing* 4, no. 4 (2007), see abstract at http://www .immunityageing.com/content/pdf/1742-4933-4-4.pdf.

5. Kevin Tracey, "Scientists Discover a Direct Route from the Brain to the Immune System," The Feinstein Institute for Medical Research, excerpt from a lecture on 10/24/07 at the NIH, see http://www.northshorelij.com/template. cfm?xyzpdqabc=0&id=204&action=detail&ref=968.

6. John McManamy, "God Power," http://www.mcmanweb.com/god_power .html.

Chapter 69 Value Yourself

1. "Self Esteem," http://en.wikipedia.org/wiki/Sel2.

2. Nathaniel Branden, *The Psychology of Self-Esteem* (Los Angeles: Nash, 1969), 252.

3. Nathaniel Branden, *The Six Pillars of Self-Esteem* (New York: Bantam, 1995), 19.

4. John M. Goldenring, MD, "How Can I Improve My Self-Esteem?" WebMD .com, http://www.webmd.com/a-to-z-guides/features/how-can-i-improve-self-esteem.

David B. Biebel, DMin, is a minister, an award-winning author, a health educator, and editor of *Today's Christian Doctor*. He often speaks on health-related subjects and has been a guest on many radio and TV programs.

He may be reached by e-mail at: DBBVI@AOL.COM. Visit his website at: http://www.crosshearthealth.com.

James E. Dill, MD, and **Bobbie Dill**, RN, were among the first husband-wife Christian medical teams to help establish a truly holistic medical practice, which they have been involved in since 1978. Jim is a board-certified gastroenterologist and Bobbie is a nurse certified in women's health. Currently they reside temporarily in various places around the United States, from Massachusetts to Hawaii, as Jim provides locum tenens medical care, often for several months at a time.